More MCQs in Cardiology for the MRCP Part 1

Presented with the compliments of Bayer plc

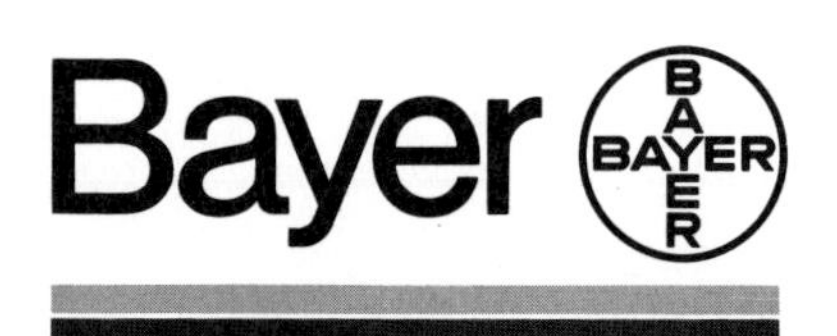

More MCQs in Cardiology for the MRCP Part 1

by

David A. Sandler, MD, MRCP
Consultant Cardiologist,
Chesterfield and North Derbyshire Royal Hospital

and

Gerald Sandler, MD, FRCP
Consultant Physician Emeritus,
Trent Regional Health Authority

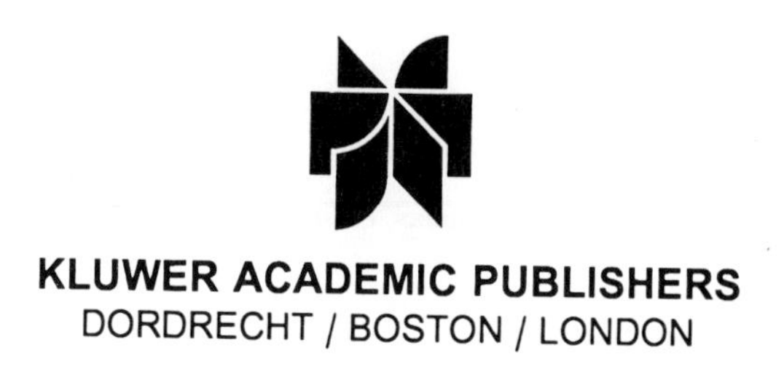

KLUWER ACADEMIC PUBLISHERS
DORDRECHT / BOSTON / LONDON

Distributors

for the United States and Canada: Kluwer Academic Publishers, PO Box 358, Accord Station, Hingham, MA 02018-0358, USA
for all other countries: Kluwer Academic Publishers Group, Distribution Center, PO Box 322, 3300 AH Dordrecht, The Netherlands

A catalogue record for this book is available from the British Library.

ISBN 0-7923-8840-2

Published in the United Kingdom by Kluwer Academic Publishers, PO Box 55, Lancaster, UK.

Kluwer Academic Publishers BV incorporates the publishing programmes of D. Reidel, Martinus Nijhoff, Dr W. Junk and MTP Press.

Printed in Great Britain by Pindar Graphics, Preston, Lancs.

Contents

Preface

Multiple choice questions are a valuable means of both acquiring knowledge and testing knowledge to see where the gaps are. They are no substitute for reading suitable cardiological texts, but they are an efficient means of determining whether what you have read has been assimilated and can be applied. Furthermore, since Part 1 of the MRCP examination includes a thorough testing of your knowledge with multiple choice questions, the more familiar you are with answering this type of question and the more practice you have had doing them, the greater your chances of passing the examination. When you have worked your way through this book, then you would be well advised to do it again until you are fully familiar with the facts in the answers, then go and look for another MCQ book of cardiological questions and work through that one also. The more you follow this procedure the greater your chances of passing what can be a difficult and searching examination.

Once again, we have tried to mix simple and more complicated topics, basic clinical examination findings and current and highly relevant research in the vanguard of cardiological treatment. We have tried to provide as much factual information and background in relation to all the possible answers offered, whether true or false. We hope it will stimulate readers to look up in more detail many of the answers we have given, which, because of the small size of this book, can necessarily be brief only. We hope that not only will the book help in the main task of passing the examination, but it will also help the reader to become a better cardiologist.

Questions

ACE INHIBITORS

1. When considering which ACE inhibitor to use: (ans. p. 35)

A. enalapril should be used if liver disease is present
B. captopril contains sulph-hydryl groups which may be responsible for its side-effects
C. captopril should not be used in diabetic patients
D. enalapril causes proteinuria and should therefore be avoided
E. a skin rash with one ACE inhibitor does not rule out the use of another

ACUTE MYOCARDIAL INFARCTION

2. The ISIS 2 Study (Second International Study of Infarct Survival, Lancet 1988;2:349–60): (ans. p. 35)

A. compared streptokinase (SK) with TPA in acute myocardial infarction
B. recruited patients up to 12 hours from onset of major symptoms
C. showed a reduction in mortality in those given aspirin alone
D. showed synergy in effect on mortality with combined therapy
E. showed a reduced mortality in patients of all ages

3. In which of the following complications is pacing of the heart required, and indicate whether the pacing should be temporary or permanent (ans. p. 36)

A. accelerated idioventricular rhythm
B. persistent first degree AV block with new bundle-branch block
C. pre-existing bifascicular block
D. Mobitz type II AV block in inferior infarction
E. marked sinus bradycardia

ANTI-ARRHYTHMIC AGENTS

4. **In using a combination of anti-arrhythmic agents:** (ans. p. 36)

A. lignocaine and β-blockers should not be administered together
B. quinidine and digoxin may be prescribed together
C. sotalol should not be combined with amiodarone
D. combinations of different Class I agents are potentially useful
E. quinidine can be given to patients on diuretics

5. **When considering the action of anti-arrhythmic medications, using the Vaughan-Williams classification:** (ans. p. 37)

A. Class IV agents alter the refractory time of the SA node
B. the Class III agents act by increasing the His–Purkinje refractory time
C. the Class II agents act predominantly on the β_2 receptors of the ventricular muscle
D. not all the Class I agents increase the refractory period of the His–Purkinje fibres
E. Class I agents inhibit the fast sodium current

AORTIC DISEASE

6. **Dissection of the aorta** (ans. p. 37)

A. is rarely associated with hypertension
B. is not due to a congenital abnormality
C. in cocaine abusers results from arterial wall damage
D. usually starts with an intimal tear in the arch of the aorta
E. is best diagnosed by CT scanning of the thorax

AORTIC REGURGITATION

7. **Aortic regurgitation** (ans. p. 38)

A. has a poor prognosis if medically treated
B. may be caused by rupture of a coronary sinus aneurysm
C. may be associated with a patent ductus in the Osler–Weber–Rendu syndrome
D. is associated with a normal ECG appearance
E. the chest X-ray does not show calcification in the aorta

AORTIC VALVE STENOSIS

8. **In a patient with aortic valve stenosis:** (ans. p. 38)

A. there is often a prominent, bifid P wave in V1 of the ECG
B. a calcified valve may be seen in younger patients above the level of the oblique fissure on a chest X-ray
C. the appearance of the valve on M-mode echocardiography does not give a good assessment of the severity of the stenosis
D. immediate valve replacement is necessary once diagnosis is made
E. of congenital origin it is often associated with coarctation of the aorta

ARRHYTHMIAS

9. **With regard to the QT interval on an ECG:** (ans. p. 39)

A. it normally shortens with exercise
B. it is normally <0.42 seconds
C. the Romano–Ward syndrome is dominantly inherited
D. the hereditary syndromes of prolongation may present as sudden death in young adults
E. hereditary prolongation can be controlled with the implantation of a permanent pacemaker

10. When considering the likely mechanisms or causes of arrhythmias: (ans. p. 39)

A. an AV re-entry circuit is the commonest mechanism for a supraventricular arrhythmia
B. a regular broad complex tachycardia is most likely to be ventricular tachycardia
C. retrograde flow through the Bundle of Kent is the cause of the tachycardia in WPW syndrome
D. sinus tachycardia is unlikely if the ventricular rate is >150/min
E. a narrow complex arrhythmia at a rate of about 150/min is likely to be atrial flutter

11. When investigating a patient for arrhythmias with a 24-hour ECG recording: (ans. p. 40)

A. evidence of heart block may be quite normal
B. tachycardia of <140/min is usually of no haemodynamic significance
C. ventricular bigeminy reduces cerebral blood flow
D. asystolic pauses may be normal
E. ventricular ectopic beats are rarely of importance

12. In the termination of a tachycardia with a pacing wire: (ans. p. 40)

A. underdrive pacing is the most effective way of abolishing a resistant tachycardia
B. overdrive pacing is of no use in ventricular arrhythmias
C. the use of an early 'extra-stimulus' is rarely useful
D. pacing wire should not be removed immediately sinus rhythm is restored
E. atrial pacing is preferable to ventricular pacing most times

13. In attempting to terminate supraventricular tachycardia (ans. p. 41)

A. ipecachuana is of no clinical use
B. the 'diving reflex' requires full immersion of the head in water
C. eyeball pressure is ineffective
D. carotid sinus massage should not be performed with the patient sitting down
E. the Valsalva manoeuvre is the most effective non-pharmacological method of terminating an arrhythmia

ARTERIAL PULSE

14. When examining the arterial pulse: (ans. p. 41)

A. an anacrotic pulse may be present in febrile states
B. a small-volume, collapsing pulse is a feature of aortic valve disease
C. a large-volume collapsing pulse is diagnostic of mitral regurgitation
D. a rise in pressure on expiration represents pericardial constriction
E. pulsus alternans represents cardiac failure

ATRIAL FIBRILLATION

15. The risk of thrombo-embolic complications in non-rheumatic atrial fibrillation: (ans. p. 42)

A. causing stroke is about 10% per year
B. is significantly reduced by warfarin
C. is higher in patients aged less than 60 years
D. is higher than the risk of serious haemorrhage on anticoagulants
E. is reduced by aspirin

16. With regard to the use of aspirin in the prevention of thrombo-embolic events in non-rheumatic atrial fibrillation: (ans. p. 42)

A. aspirin is of no benefit at a daily dose of 75 mg
B. aspirin is of benefit at a daily dose of 325 mg
C. the benefits of aspirin are comparable to those of warfarin
D. aspirin is useful in patients unable to take warfarin safely
E. aspirin gives rise to significantly more haemorrhagic events than placebo

ATRIAL NATRIURETIC FACTOR

17. Atrial natriuretic factor (ANF): (ans. p. 42)

A. is produced solely in the left atrium
B. is always elevated in the blood in heart failure, irrespective of whether it is left or right ventricular failure
C. blood level is dependent on the sodium intake
D. rises with effective diuretic treatment of the heart failure
E. secretion causes an increase in blood pressure

AUSCULTATION OF THE HEART

18. When listening to added sounds on auscultation of the heart: (ans. p. 43)

A. the third heart sound is due to ventricular filling during early diastole
B. a fourth heart sound is not a feature of atrial fibrillation
C. a gallop rhythm is rare in normal hearts after the age of 30
D. a third heart sound is present in hypertension
E. a third sound is of no significance in patients under the age of 30

19. When auscultating the second heart sound: (ans. p. 43)

A. aortic valve closure precedes pulmonary closure
B. the two components are widely split in aortic stenosis
C. the second sound usually appears fixed and split in atrial septal defects
D. an absent second sound may indicate coarctation of the aorta
E. it may be palpable in transposition of the great vessels

BETA-BLOCKERS

20. When using β-blockers for cardiac disease: (ans. p. 44)

A. they may be used in diabetics
B. they may be used in patients with Raynaud's phenomenon
C. they may not be used in co-existent liver disease
D. they may not be given to patients about to undergo surgery
E. they should not be given to asthmatic patients

21. In using β-blockers in clinical practice: (ans. p. 44)

A. they can be used in all forms of angina
B. they should not be combined with calcium antagonists in treating angina
C. they should not be first-line therapy for elderly patients with hypertension
D. young, non-smoking hypertensives are best started on β-blockers
E. propranolol is the preferred β-blocker for hypertension

22. When considering the side-effects of β-blockers: (ans. p. 45)

A. withdrawal from therapy because of side-effects is commoner with propranolol than atenolol
B. heart failure induced by therapy is rare in practice
C. β-blockers may aggravate hypertension by causing vasospasm
D. pindolol causes a greater fall in cardiac output than other β-blockers
E. pindolol and propranolol both cause dreams by their lipid-solubility and CNS penetration

23. In using a combination of β-blockers with other medication: (ans. p. 46)

A. β-blockers should be avoided in hypertensive patients on clonidine
B. β-blockers may be combined with reserpine in the treatment of hypertension
C. cimetidine may reduce the effects of propranolol
D. β-blockers can usefully be combined with nifedipine in hypertension and angina
E. non-steroidal anti-inflammatory drugs (NSAIDs) should not be combined with β-blockers

24. When considering whether to use a β-blocker or a calcium antagonist in the treatment of hypertension, the decision may be influenced by the following: (ans. p. 46)

A. asthmatic patients can safely receive either
B. neither calcium-channel blockers nor β-blockers alter the lipid profile unfavourably
C. not all calcium-channel blockers aggravate cardiac failure by their negative inotropism
D. verapamil is relatively safe in digitalis toxicity
E. diltiazem should be avoided in obstructive cardiomyopathy

25. In using β-blockers (ans. p. 47)

A. their anti-arrhythmic properties are due to shortening of the action-potential in cardiac cells
B. β-blockers with intrinsic sympathomimetic activity (ISA) improve sleep patterns
C. atenolol is the most cardio-selective β-blocker and therefore best for asthmatic patients requiring these agents
D. if β-blockers are essential in patients with airway obstruction, a cardio-selective drug is preferable to a β-blocker with high intrinsic sympathomimetic activity
E. combined α- and β-blockade by labetalol is more effective in hypertension than propranolol

CARDIAC AND BRONCHIAL ASTHMA

26. In differentiating acute dyspnoea caused by LV failure (LVF) from that due to bronchial asthma (BA): (ans. p. 47)

A. loud diffuse wheezing favours BA
B. the patient with LVF sweats profusely while in BA the skin is dry
C. a gallop rhythm is a very helpful sign
D. if the patient has Curschmann's sign this is diagnostic of LVF
E. cyanosis favours LVF

CARDIAC ARRHYTHMIAS

27. A Stokes–Adams attack: (ans. p. 48)

A. is rarely preceded by an aura
B. may be precipitated by a grand-mal convulsion
C. is associated with flushing at the time of collapse
D. normal consciousness slowly returns once the circulation is restored
E. usually results in prolonged unconsciousness

CARDIAC DRUGS

28. With regard to the use of sodium nitroprusside in cardiac failure and cardiogenic shock: (ans. p. 48)

A. a hypothyroid state may be induced
B. should be administered with a concurrent dose of thiamine
C. the infusion is nephrotoxic
D. free cyanide is predominantly erythrocyte-bound before excretion
E. the metabolite is renally excreted

CARDIAC GLYCOSIDES

29. When using cardiac glycosides: (ans. p. 49)

A. ouabain acts rapidly when administered intravenously or orally
B. digitoxin is disadvantageous as it has a long half-life
C. lantoside C differs from digoxin only in its side-effect profile
D. intravenous digoxin acts significantly more quickly than an orally administered dose
E. digoxin has a long half-life and remains the preferred glycoside

CARDIAC SURGERY

30. When considering patients with prosthetic valves: (ans. p. 49)

A. tilting disc valves have a shorter life than silastic ball valves
B. warfarin in unnecessary for all mechanical valves
C. tissue valves give rise to structural failure many years after implantation
D. endocarditis is commoner in the aortic position
E. haemolysis is a frequent complication

CARDIAC THERAPY

31. Precautions necessary when starting treatment with ACE inhibitors include: (ans. p. 50)

A. using a small test-dose first
B. monitor serum potassium level daily
C. a renal angiogram is advisable before treatment is started
D. hospital admission is not essential
E. reduce diuretics 24 to 48 hours before initiating therapy

CARDIAC TRANSPLANTATION

32. Cardiac transplantation: (ans. p. 50)

A. is usually complicated by episodes of rejection
B. can be performed effectively in the presence of pulmonary hypertension
C. no longer requires lifelong immunosuppression
D. is rarely complicated by bacterial infection
E. is usually followed by atheroma in the donor heart

CARDIAC TRAUMA

33. External cardiac trauma: (ans. p. 51)

A. may be a precursor of angina
B. commonly causes pericardial damage and pericarditis
C. may cause mitral incompetence
D. when it causes death from cardiac complications, the commonest cause of death is myocardial infarction
E. can be easily diagnosed from blood levels of cardiac enzymes

CHOLESTEROL AND HEART DISEASE

34. Is it true or false that: (ans. p. 51)

A. lowering the blood cholesterol may increase mortality from coronary heart disease
B. lowering blood cholesterol increases the incidence of bowel cancer
C. the increased mortality found in cholesterol-lowering trials is attributable to causes other than organic disease
D. variation in levels of blood cholesterol can directly affect brain function
E. cholesterol-lowering drugs vary in their potential to cause increased mortality

CHRONIC CONSTRICTIVE PERICARDITIS

35. Chronic constrictive pericarditis: (ans. p. 52)

A. in current practice is rarely caused by tuberculosis
B. is frequently associated with a pulsus paradoxus
C. can be differentiated from restrictive cardiomyopathy by detecting left ventricular insufficiency as well as right ventricular dysfunction
D. is best treated surgically
E. is equally frequent in men and women

CLINICAL EXAMINATION

36. The apex beat: (ans. p. 52)

A. normally lifts the examining finger off the chest
B. will be thrusting in aortic regurgitation
C. is hyperdynamic and laterally displaced in a VSD
D. is not palpable in a perfectly normal person
E. may feel like a double impulse in hypertension

CONGENITAL HEART BLOCK

37. Which of the following are likely to be true in complete heart block of congenital origin? (ans. p. 53)

A. the prognosis is poorer if the condition is familial
B. the haemodynamic response to exercise is normal
C. it is rarely associated with other serious cardiac arrhythmias
D. it may follow connective tissue disease in the mother
E. pregnancy is contraindicated in women with congenital complete heart block

38. Which of the following statements are true? (ans. p. 53)

A. most infants with CHB have associated cardiac abnormalities
B. maternal disease can cause CHB in the infant
C. the condition carries a good prognosis
D. there are serious risks if a patient with CHB becomes pregnant
E. the condition occurs predominantly in male infants

CONGENITAL HEART DISEASE

39. When considering patients with congenital heart disease: (ans. p. 54)

A. the incidence is about 8 per 1000 live births
B. a ventricular septal defect is the most common congenital heart lesion
C. spontaneous closure of a VSD occurs in <10% patients
D. ASD results in pulmonary hypertension
E. patent ductus arteriosus and VSD usually co-exist

CORONARY ARTERY DISEASE

40. **In coronary artery spasm:** (ans. p. 54)

A. there may not be a resultant tachycardia
B. there is an increase in end-diastolic intraventricular pressure
C. coronary arteriography is rarely normal
D. the aetiological factor is an abnormality of collagen in the coronary artery walls
E. myocardial oxygen supply is reduced before the episode of chest pain

DIGOXIN

41. **Digoxin:** (ans. p. 55)

A. is quickly absorbed after oral administration
B. is lipid soluble
C. is not strongly bound to plasma proteins
D. is metabolised in the liver before excretion
E. may be poorly absorbed in hypothyroidism

DISSECTION OF THE AORTA

42. **Dissection of the aorta:** (ans. p. 55)

A. has a mortality of about 30%
B. death results from cardiac tamponade in fatal cases
C. should not be treated with hypotensive medication
D. must usually be treated by surgery
E. may be complicated by myocardial infarction

DRIVING REGULATIONS AND CARDIOVASCULAR DISEASE

43. The following cardiovascular conditions, if present, always disqualify the patient from holding a PSV or HGV licence (ans. p. 56)

A. dissection of the aorta
B. dilatation of the aortic root
C. an episode of unstable angina
D. angina and an aortic aneurysm
E. intermittent claudication

44. A PSV/HGV licence will not be allowed in the following circumstances: (ans. p. 56)

A. treated hypertension
B. severe hypertension
C. treated arrhythmia
D. a pacemaker is fitted
E. a cardioverter/defibrillator is fitted

45. Regarding an HGV/PSV licence, a coronary angiogram: (ans. p. 56)

A. is necessary after a myocardial infarction if a PSV/HGV licence is to be reinstated
B. showing an ejection fraction of >30% is permissible for the return of the PSV/HGV licence
C. showing any significant occlusion of a major coronary artery will be a bar to regaining a licence
D. demonstrating 2-vessel disease disqualifies the holder
E. must be normal before the licence can be returned

46. A person may not hold a PSV/HGV licence if: (ans. p. 57)

A. he has ever had a myocardial infarction
B. he has had coronary angioplasty
C. he cannot reach the end of Stage IV of the Bruce protocol on a treadmill
D. he develops ventricular tachycardia during exercise
E. he has coronary artery disease and has not had an angiogram

DRUG THERAPY IN HEART DISEASE

47. With regard to the use of vasodilator therapy: (ans. p. 57)

A. isosorbide infusions are potent venous dilators
B. nitroprusside is a mixed venous and arterial vasodilator
C. salbutamol infusions may induce hypokalaemia
D. nitroprusside infusions may cause a metabolic acidosis if continued beyond 48 hours
E. hydrallazine therapy causes venodilatation and a fall in venous return

EBSTEIN'S ANOMALY

48. Which of the following statements are true? (ans. p. 57)

A. in Ebstein's anomaly the right ventricular papillary muscle is usually normal. The main abnormality is malinsertion of the tricuspid valve so that the proximal part of the right ventricle is incorporated into the atrium
B. pulmonary regurgitation may be associated with Ebstein's anomaly in symptomatic infants. An atrial septal defect is present in most cases
C. on auscultation there is splitting of both first and second heart sounds
D. the ECG is usually non-specific and not very helpful in diagnosis
E. cardiac catheterisation may be diagnostic

ECG

49. **The causes of an increased R wave in lead V1 of the ECG include:** (ans. p. 58)

A. Wolff–Parkinson–White syndrome
B. postero-inferior myocardial infarction
C. left anterior hemiblock
D. left posterior hemiblock without myocardial infarction
E. hyperkalaemia

50. **When studying the ECG:** (ans. p. 58)

A. a cardiac axis of >-30 degrees represents left axis deviation
B. right axis deviation is not associated with a secundum ASD
C. left axis deviation commonly coexists with an ostium primum atrial septal defect
D. right bundle branch block is a sign of block in the posterior hemi-bundle
E. pulmonary stenosis may cause axis deviation

FIBRINOLYTIC THERAPY

51. **The ASSET study (Anglo Scandinavian Study of Early Thrombolysis):** (ans. p. 59)

A. compared tissue plasminogen activator (TPA) to placebo in acute myocardial infarction
B. did not require anticoagulation post thrombolysis
C. confirmed a reduction in mortality after fibrinolysis
D. showed that only patients with ECG changes at entry had a reduced mortality
E. showed an increase incidence of haemorrhagic stroke in those given TPA.

52. **With regard to heparin therapy after fibrinolytic administration:** (ans. p. 59)

A. heparin should never be used after fibrinolytics
B. heparin increases platelet activation
C. heparin reduces the incidence of re-thrombosis
D. heparin induces platelet thrombosis
E. heparin inhibits fibrin formation on platelet surfaces

HEART MURMURS

53. **Innocent heart murmurs:** (ans. p. 60)

A. are common in younger patients
B. are usually systolic
C. are associated with other abnormal sounds
D. are heard at the left sternal edge
E. require investigation

HYPERTENSION

54. **Which of the following hypotensive drugs should be avoided in hypertensive patients with the conditions listed below (more than one answer for each condition is acceptable when appropriate)** (ans. p. 60)

A. diuretic
B. β-blocker
C. ACE inhibitor
D. calcium-channel blocker
E. α-blocker

1. renal artery stenosis
2. gout
3. asthma
4. heart failure
5. diabetes

55. Select the hypotensive drug group (A–E below) which has the side-effect profile tabulated below (1–5 in table): (ans. p. 60)

A. diuretic
B. β-blocker
C. ACE inhibitor
D. calcium channel blocker
E. α-blocker

Profile	*1*	*2*	*3*	*4*	*5*
headache	–	+	–	–	–
flushing	–	+	–	–	–
dyspnoea	–	–	–	–	+
lethargy	–	–	–	–	+
impotence	–	–	+	–	+
cough	+	–	–	–	–
gout	–	–	+	–	–
oedema	–	+	–	–	–
postural hypotension	–	–	+	+	–
cold extremities	–	–	–	–	+

56. The British Hypertension Society, in its recently published guidance on the management of hypertension (Br Med J. 1993;306:983), recommend the following for the correct measurement of blood pressure: (ans. p. 61)

A. patient should be lying on a couch
B. record pressure to the nearest 5 mm mercury
C. take 4 measurements over 4 visits before diagnosing hypertension
D. standing BP to be taken in elderly patients
E. check BP over 3 to 6 months before treating

57. The British Hypertension Society, in its recently published guidance on the management of hypertension (Br Med J. 1993;306:983), recommend the following: (ans. p. 61)

A. patients aged 68–80 should not be treated unless their systolic BP is persistently over 200 mm
B. patients aged 60–80 do not require treatment if diastolic pressures are <90 mm
C. hypotensive therapy should not be started in the over 80s
D. isolated systolic hypertension requires no treatment if the diastolic pressure is below 90 mm
E. treatment should be withdrawn if the diastolic pressure is persistently <80 mm and the systolic <160

INFECTIVE ENDOCARDITIS

58. Which of the following statements are true about infective endocarditis: (ans. p. 61)

A. it usually affects a previously abnormal heart valve
B. *Streptococcus pneumoniae* is the putative infecting agent in most cases
C. infections with multiple organisms are rarely seen in drug addicts
D. it should initially be treated with at least 2 antibiotics
E. it rarely requires 6 weeks of intravenous antibiotics

INOTROPIC SYMPATHOMIMETIC MEDICATION

59. When considering the use of inotropic sympathomimetic medication: (ans. p. 62)

A. noradrenaline causes intense vasodilatation
B. isoprenaline causes a β-receptor-mediated tachycardia
C. dopamine causes the release of noradrenaline from the heart
D. dopamine is a peripheral vasodilator
E. dobutamine predominantly stimulates β_2 receptors

INSULIN AND HEART DISEASE

60. In the relationship between insulin and atherosclerosis, which of the following statements are true? (ans. p. 62)

A. the level of circulating blood insulin is related to the risk of developing atherosclerosis
B. insulin has a direct action on the arterial wall
C. patients with hyperinsulinaemia tend to have lower blood pressure than normal
D. insulin treatment of diabetic patients increases the incidence of coronary disease
E. the use of nicotinic acid as a cholesterol-lowering drug increases mortality in patients with previous myocardial infarction, because it causes hyperinsulinaemia

MARFAN SYNDROME

61. Marfan syndrome: (ans. p. 63)

A. is equally common in males and females
B. may sometimes occur in the absence of any cardiac involvement
C. the primary cardiac involvement is in the aorta and the mitral valve is never affected
D. may sometimes cause blue sclerae
E. the cardiac complications may be favorably influenced by drug treatment

MATERNAL MORTALITY DUE TO HEART DISEASE IN PREGNANCY

62. Which of the following statements are true or false? (ans. p. 64)

A. heart disease is now the commonest cause of maternal mortality in the UK. The death rate is remaining relatively constant since the early seventies – about 1 death per 100,000 live births
B. the most recent report of national maternal mortality statistics [1] showed that the incidence of acquired heart disease is increasing
C. when maternal death is due to acquired heart disease, the commonest cause is valvular heart disease
D. puerperal cardiomyopathy still remains a serious hazard in spite of modern treatment
E. anticoagulants should not be used at any time when treating patients with puerperal cardiomyopathy

[1] DHSS report on confidential enquiries and maternal deaths in England and Wales 1983–87. HMSO 1991.

METABOLIC HEART DISEASE

63. Which of the following statements are true? (ans. p. 64)

A. cardiomyopathy may be a complication of phaeochromocytoma
B. Wolff–Parkinson–White syndrome may occur in glycogen-storage disease
C. infants born of mothers with beri-beri may also develop cardiomyopathy due to vitamin B1 deficiency
D. the commonest cause of death in haemachromatosis is congestive cardiac failure
E. diabetic mothers never produce babies with diabetic cardiomyopathy

MITRAL REGURGITATION

64. **In mitral regurgitation:** (ans. p. 65)

A. the murmur may be loudest at the apex
B. the murmur is loudest in the back if the anterior chordae have ruptured
C. the best view of mitral regurgitation at catheter is in the right anterior oblique position
D. the appearance of the 'v' wave at cardiac catheter is unrelated to the severity of the regurgitation
E. there is a poor prognosis in the presence of good LV function

MITRAL STENOSIS

65. **Mitral stenosis:** (ans. p. 65)

A. may be a congenital lesion of the heart
B. most commonly follows an infection with a group A streptococcal organism
C. is best differentiated from an atrial myxoma simulating mitral stenosis by echocardiography
D. is characterised by fatigue, which may be the presenting symptom
E. may be associated with dysphagia

66. **In mitral stenosis:** (ans. p. 66)

A. the degree of stenosis of the valve is reflected in the loudness of the murmur
B. the position of the opening snap in the cardiac cycle is unrelated to the severity of stenosis
C. more severe stenosis causes longer diastolic murmurs
D. is often associated with a third heart sound
E. is rarely associated with chronic bronchitis

MITRAL VALVE SYNDROME

67. The floppy mitral valve syndrome (mitral valve prolapse): (ans. p. 66)

A. occurs in about 5% of the normal, asymptomatic population
B. usually involves one of the leaflets of the valve and the chordae
C. exhibits an impulse suggesting a double apex beat
D. is responsible for the 3rd heart sound that is present on auscultation
E. the murmur becomes louder after amyl nitrite, which distinguishes it from hypertrophic obstructive cardiomyopathy, which has a similar murmur

MYOCARDIAL INFARCTION

68. The ST segment depression seen in the ECG leads other than those subtending the area of acute myocardial infarction (ans. p. 67)

A. represents other ischaemic areas
B. is not a reflection of the size of the infarction
C. identifies coronary artery disease in other sites
D. identifies patients at higher risk of complications
E. bears little relationship to findings on exercise testing

69. For the major trials of fibrinolytic therapy in acute myocardial infarction listed below, all of which showed a reduction in mortality in treated patients compared to controls, attempt to match the therapy used and the time after symptom onset that allowed patient inclusion: (ans. p. 67)

1. GISSI Lancet. 1987;1:392
2. ISAM N Engl J Med. 1986;314:1465–71
3. ISIS 2 Lancet. 1988;2:349–60
4. AIMS Lancet. 1988;1:545–9
5. ASSET Lancet. 1988;2:525–30

	Fibrinolytic drug		*Time to inclusion*
A.	Streptokinase	(i)	<5 hours
B.	Tissue plasminogen activator	(ii)	<6 hours
C.	Anisoylated streptokinase plasminogen complex	(iii)	<12 hours
		(iv)	<24 hours

70. **Subendocardial myocardial infarction:** (ans. p. 67)

A. results in changes to the QRS complexes on the ECG
B. may follow a transmural infarction
C. is unrelated to coronary vascular resistance
D. is not caused by valvular heart disease
E. may be related to successful resuscitation from cardiac arrest

71. **When myocardial infarction occurs in an elderly patient:** (ans. p. 68)

A. chest pain is usually the presenting complaint
B. 'silent infarction' is unusual
C. it is often associated with severe dyspnoea in the absence of acute LVF
D. it is associated with a higher mortality
E. there is little to be gained from fibrinolytic therapy

72. **Right ventricular infarction:** (ans. p. 69)

A. is a common pathological finding at autopsy
B. is diagnosed on the ECG by ST elevation in lead V1R
C. may result in cardiogenic shock
D. associated with cardiac failure will improve on diuretics
E. has clinical findings similar to those of left ventricular failure

73. Pericardial effusion after a myocardial infarction: (ans. p. 69)

A. is a rare complication
B. is not associated with an increased mortality
C. resolves slowly without treatment
D. is only one cause of a posterior echo-free space on echocardiography
E. is unrelated to the healing that follows the infarction

74. In acute myocardial infarction: (ans. p. 70)

A. thrombotic occlusion precedes plaque rupture
B. the initiating event is platelet activation
C. total occlusion of the infarct-related artery may result in non-Q-wave infarction
D. thrombolytic therapy has no effect on the arterial lumen
E. injury deep in the arterial wall induces thrombosis

MYOCARDITIS

75. In patients with myocarditis: (ans. p. 70)

A. a bacterial aetiology is usual
B. general viral infections are often associated with cardiac involvement
C. females are affected more than males
D. the ECG is rarely diagnostic
E. treatment with immunosuppressives should not be administered

NITRATES

76. **In using nitrates:** (ans. p. 71)

A. dinitrates offer advantages over mononitrates
B. the nitrate patch has little benefit over oral agents
C. nitrates act in angina mainly by reducing coronary spasm
D. their vasodilatory actions are beneficial in cardiac failure
E. they may be less effective in angina as double-therapy with a β-blocker or calcium antagonist, than triple-therapy with both additional drugs

77. **Nitrates:** (ans. p. 71)

A. are contraindicated in the treatment of angina associated with hypertrophic obstructive cardiomyopathy
B. are indicated in constrictive pericarditis
C. may be safely prescribed in anterior myocardial infarction
D. must not be given to patients with glaucoma
E. are not associated with a significant withdrawal syndrome

78. **Which of the following are true or false?** (ans. p. 72)

A. nitrates should not be used for treating patients with severe left ventricular failure if the patient is already taking hydralazine
B. nitrates are contraindicated in end-stage renal failure
C. nitrates are effective in the treatment of angina associated with hypertrophic obstructive cardiomyopathy (HOCM)
D. nitrates should not be used in constrictive pericarditis
E. nitrates are contraindicated in glaucoma

PAROXYSMAL ATRIAL FIBRILLATION (PAF)

79. Indicate whether true or false? (ans. p. 72)

A. the incidence of thrombo-embolism is similar in PAF and sustained AF
B. digoxin is an effective treatment in prevention of attacks
C. verapamil has little effect in controlling PAF
D. when PAF is a manifestation of sick-sinus syndrome, the best treatment is simple ventricular pacing
E. amiodarone is the drug of choice

PERCUTANEOUS, TRANSLUMINAL CORONARY ANGIOPLASTY

80. The procedure: (ans. p. 73)

A. is unlikely to restenose after 6 months
B. is frequently associated with occlusion during the procedure
C. need not be restricted to single vessel disease
D. may be attempted across bypass grafts which have stenosed
E. should not be carried out in the X-ray department of most district general hospitals

POST-MYOCARDIAL INFARCTION

81. In assessing the post-myocardial infarction syndrome: (ans. p. 74)

A. the diagnoses of shoulder–hand syndrome and Dressler syndrome are synonymous
B. the shoulder–hand syndrome affects the left upper limb only
C. Dupuytren's contracture can sometimes occur in the shoulder–hand syndrome
D. Dressler syndrome is an auto-immune disease
E. Dressler beats are one of the diagnostic features of Dressler syndrome

82. In trials of β-blockers after acute myocardial infarction: (ans. p. 74)

A. effects are mediated through their anti-arrhythmic action
B. the Norwegian study confirmed the value of metoprolol
C. propranolol has been shown to be of value
D. early administration of atenolol increases early deaths
E. treatment should be continued for 2 years

POST-MYOCARDIAL INFARCTION PROPHYLAXIS

83. In secondary prevention after myocardial infarction: (ans. p. 75)

A. anticoagulation with warfarin is of proven value
B. aspirin is of proven value
C. dipyridamole is of no proven value as sole therapy
D. antiarrhythmics have been shown to be of value
E. sulphinpyrazone prolongs survival

PRIMARY PULMONARY HYPERTENSION (PPH)

84. Which of the following statements are true in PPH? (ans. p. 75)

A. PPH affects males and females equally
B. infection can play a significant part in its aetiology
C. Raynaud disease is common in patients with PPH
D. PPH is caused mainly by recurrent pulmonary thrombo-embolic disease
E. diagnosis is made by ventilation/perfusion lung scan

QT SYNDROME

85. In the prolonged QT syndrome: (ans. p. 76)

A. the duration of the QT interval depends on the heart rate
B. the effect of exercise is to shorten the QT interval
C. it can sometimes be associated with deafness
D. hyperkalaemia makes the condition worse
E. the cause may be dietary irregularities

RADIATION AND HEART DISEASE

86. Which of the following are true? (ans. p. 76)

A. the heart is a relatively radio-resistant organ
B. if the heart is affected by radiation it is usually the heart valves which are damaged most
C. myocardial infarction does not occur as a complication of radiation therapy
D. in treating breast cancer by DXR the development of cardiac complications does not depend on which side the breast cancer is present
E. when the coronary arteries are affected by DXR they are all equally involved

RHEUMATIC FEVER

87. Match the incidence figures of the following complications of acute rheumatic fever: (ans. p. 87)

Complication
A. carditis
B. arthritis
C. chorea (St Vitus Dance)
D. permanent valvular disease
E. erythema marginatum

Incidence (a) 80% (b) 50% (c) 10% (d) 5% (e) 30%

RHEUMATOID HEART DISEASE

88. In rheumatoid heart disease as opposed to rheumatic heart disease: (ans. p. 77)

A. myocarditis is unlikely to occur
B. if pericarditis occurs it is usually 'dry'
C. the mitral valve is the valve most likely to be affected
D. the commonest ECG abnormality is left bundle branch block
E. coronary artery disease is common

SARCOIDOSIS AND THE HEART

89. Which statements are true? (ans. p. 77)

A. heart failure is the commonest cause of death in patients with sarcoidosis in the UK
B. the commonest clinical presentation is heart block
C. anginal pain rarely occurs in sarcoidosis
D. endomyocardial diagnosis is almost invariably positive in myocardial sarcoidosis
E. steroids should be used with caution in treating a patient with sarcoidosis and cardiac involvement

SYMPATHOMIMETICS

90. Dobutamine: (ans. p. 78)

A. administration must be carried out through a peripheral vein
B. has no dopaminergic effect on the heart
C. causes the release of adrenaline within the circulation
D. has a marked chronotropic effect at therapeutic doses
E. is a peripheral vasoconstrictor

TAKAYASU'S ARTERITIS

91. Takayasu's arteritis: (ans. p. 79)

A. the cause is auto-immune disease
B. the sexes are equally affected
C. was first diagnosed on ophthalmological examination
D. is never associated with pulmonary artery involvement
E. can only be distinguished from coarctation of the aorta by angiography

VENTRICULAR ANEURYSM

92. Which of the following statements are true? (ans. p. 79)

A. ventricular aneurysm never occurs as a result of non-ischaemic heart disease
B. following myocardial infarction left ventricular aneurysm occurs equally in the front and the back of the heart
C. the development of a left ventricular aneurysm is related to the extent of the coronary vessel involvement
D. true ventricular aneurysms are unlikely to rupture
E. ventricular aneurysm is one of the most common causes of heart failure in coronary heart disease

VENTRICULAR SEPTAL DEFECT

93. Ventricular septal defect after myocardial infarction: (ans. p. 80)

A. rarely affects the anterior or apical segment of the septum
B. rarely involves the mitral valve
C. is never followed by a septal aneurysm
D. usually occurs within the first three days
E. is usually associated with a significant increase in mortality

VENTRICULAR TACHYCARDIA

94. Ventricular tachycardia: (ans. p. 80)

A. may not require treatment in all circumstances
B. requires DC shock in almost all cases
C. is associated with hyperkalaemia
D. should not be treated with bretylium tosylate
E. of the torsades de pointes variety is best treated by non-pharmacological means

95. In the differentiation between ventricular tachycardia and supraventricular tachycardia with aberrant conduction: (ans. p. 81)

A. an atrial electrogram is unlikely to be helpful
B. the presence of pre-existing bundle branch block is of no diagnostic value
C. an Rsr pattern in V1 on the ECG favours an atrial origin to the tachycardia
D. the deepest QS wave appears in V1–3 in ventricular tachycardia
E. changing wave fronts should lead to a diagnosis of VT

Answers

ACE INHIBITORS

1.

A – **F** it is metabolised in the liver and should be avoided in patients with liver cell impairment; captopril may be better as it does not undergo liver metabolism

B – **T** it is thought that these may be responsible for some of its toxic side-effects such as the rash, taste disturbance and proteinuria. Enalapril does not contain such groups and may therefore have fewer of these side-effects

C – **F** captopril may be of some benefit if patients with diabetic nephropathy have proteinuria; the reasons for this benefit are unknown

D – **F** enalapril may reduce the creatinine clearance in patients with congestive cardiac failure, but does not cause proteinuria; captopril, however, does lead to proteinuria in high doses and renal function should therefore be monitored carefully

E – **T** patients who have had a skin rash with captopril have been safely given enalapril

ACUTE MYOCARDIAL INFARCTION

2.

A – **F** ISIS 2 compared 1.5 megaUnits SK infused over 1 hour and/or 160 mg aspirin/day for 1 month (or identical placebos) in >17,000 patients presenting within 24 hours of an acute myocardial infarction

B – **F** patients were recruited up to 24 hours after onset of their major symptoms

C – **T** aspirin alone reduced mortality by 25% at 5 weeks from 12% to 9.2%

D – **T** there was a mortality reduction on combined therapy of 42%; from 13.2% to 8%

E – **T** treatment was equally effective in the 20% of trial patients over the age of 70 years, and this improved mortality was maintained at up to 15 months after infarction

3. A this condition occurs mainly with inferior infarction. Pacing is not required as it is almost invariably transient and is very rarely associated with any further development of heart block

B this condition requires permanent pacing as survivors of myocardial infarction with these complications have a high incidence of recurrent high-degree AV block and sudden death

C if the duration of the bifascicular block is known and the condition is stable, pacing is not required. However, if the duration of the block is unknown or new first-degree block occurs with the infarction, then temporary pacing is desirable

D temporary pacing is indicated as some of these patients may go on to symptomatic complete heart block

E if the sinus bradycardia is asymptomatic, even though marked, then pacing is not required. The presence of angina, left ventricular failure or syncope requires temporary pacing

ANTI-ARRHYTHMIC AGENTS

4. A – **T** β-blockers will result in reduced hepatic clearance of lignocaine and therefore increase the tendency to side-effects

B – **F** there is displacement of digoxin from protein-bound sites in patients on quinidine, increased blood digoxin levels and therefore an increased tendency to digoxin toxicity

C – **T** the combination of more than one Class III agent increases the likelihood of a prolonged QT interval which in turn encourages 'torsades de pointes' ventricular tachycardia

D – **F** each Class I drug may cause depression, both of conduction and also myocardial contractility because of the negative inotropic property of this class of drug

E – **F** diuretic-induced hypokalaemia may increase the risk of 'torsades de pointes'

5.

A – **F** Class IV agents, the calcium antagonists, act by increasing the duration of AV node refractoriness

B – **T** Class III drugs (e.g. amiodarone and sotalol) increase the time taken for His–Purkinje fibres to undergo further depolarisation and so reduce the ventricular response

C – **F** Class II agents, the β-blockers, primarily depress the sinus node and the AV node and have little direct action on the ventricular muscle through their β-receptors

D – **T** although Class Ia (e.g. procainamide and disopyramide) and Ic agents (e.g. flecainide, propafenone) do increase the refractory period, Class Ib agents (e.g. lignocaine and mexilitene) actually reduce the refractoriness of the His–Purkinje fibres

E – **T** by inhibiting the fast inward sodium current, the upstroke of the action potential is inhibited and this delays the return of excitability

AORTIC DISEASE

6.

A – **F** this is the most common co-existing factor (in 30–50%) and it probably accelerates the normal process of degeneration in the smooth muscle cells of the media and the elastic tissue

B – **T** but it is associated with many congenital conditions, particularly those which affect the ascending aorta, e.g. Marfan disease, bicuspid aortic valve, coarctation

C – **F** it is due to the paroxysmal hypertension which occurs with this

D – **F** two-thirds start with an intimal tear in the ascending aorta, possibly because of repeated flexion of the aorta during systole, combined with the force of blood being ejected against the intima at the same site

E – **T** although digital subtraction angiogram, magnetic resonance imaging and transoesophageal echo are all also useful and supersede aortography, previously regarded as the 'gold standard'

AORTIC REGURGITATION

7.

A – **T** once symptoms occur and cardiomegaly is present on the chest X-ray, prognosis is poor – the 3-year survival rate is only 65%

B – **F** aortic regurgitation may result from an aneurysm of the sinus of Valsalva rupturing

C – **F** the Osler–Weber–Rendu syndrome may occasionally present with aortic regurgitation as well as cyanosis, bronchiectasis and secondary polycythaemia and a pulmonary AV fistula

D – **F** the ECG may show left ventricular hypertrophy and a 'diastolic overload' pattern of prominent Q waves in the anterolateral leads. As the condition deteriorates, ST depression and T-wave inversion occur

E – **F** if the cause of the aortic regurgitation is syphylitic then the valve will be calcified. Calcification of the aortic valve in rheumatic or congenital aortic regurgitation is rare

AORTIC VALVE STENOSIS

8.

A – **F** the P wave may be negative. Due to increased left ventricular end diastolic pressure, the P wave is an exaggeration of its usual inverted position – inverted as it is 'looking' at the heart from the right ventricular aspect

B – **T** the calcified aortic valve is above and anterior to the oblique fissure on the lateral chest X-ray

C – **T** M-mode echo is not reliable. Doppler gives a better idea of the degree of stenosis but the best method of assessment is direct measurement of the gradient across the aortic valve at catheterisation

D – **F** the onset of symptoms is the time for surgery: the average survival is only 2–3 years with angina/syncope and only 18 months once cardiac failure has occurred

E – **T** the commonest associations are with coarctation of the aorta (in Turner's syndrome) or with coarctation and a patent ductus arteriosus occurring together

ARRHYTHMIAS

9. A – **F** it is prolonged due to both increased heart rate and increased catecholamine production on exertion

B – **T** and should be corrected for heart rate (QTc) by dividing the measured interval by the square root of the cycle length

C – **T** the Romano–Ward syndrome is dominantly inherited. It is the Lange–Neilson hereditary syndrome that is recessively inherited and is associated with nerve deafness

D – **T** because of a tendency to develop ventricular tachycardia on emotion or exercise. This results in syncope and sometimes death

E – **F** as the cause is thought to be an imbalance between the sympathetic innervation on the right and left sides of the heart, full β-blockade may be effective in controlling symptoms

10. A – **T** the usual mechanism is a re-entry circuit, either within the AV node or incorporating an accessory pathway

B – **T** it is safest to assume that any broad complex tachycardia is ventricular until proven otherwise, especially in any patient with a background of ischaemic heart disease

C – **T** the supraventricular tachycardia of WPW is caused by the re-entry of an impulse, conducted antegradely through the normal AV node and then retrogradely back up the accessory bundle into the atrium. The less common fast atrial fibrillation sometimes seen with WPW is due to rapid antegrade flow through the Bundle of Kent

D – **T** a regular tachycardia of up to 150/min may be a sinus tachycardia but rates higher than this are due to SVT

E – **T** if a patient has a regular tachycardia with a rate of around 140–155, consider atrial flutter with 2:1 block

11. A – **T** first-degree block and Wenchebach AV block (in patients with high vagal tone) have been reported in normal individuals

B – **T** if the heart is otherwise normal, it is the heart rates >140/min or <40/min that are likely to decrease cerebral blood flow and therefore be responsible for symptoms

C – **T** cerebral blood flow is likely to be reduced by >10% and even this may be poorly tolerated in an elderly patient

D – **F** pauses of >2 seconds should be viewed with caution as they carry an adverse prognosis for sudden death

E – **F** frequently seen in apparently normal people, but if their frequency is >10/min they are associated with a poor prognosis in patients recovering from a myocardial infarction – there is an increased incidence of sudden death in such patients

12. A – **F** fixed-rate pacing at a rate slower than the tachycardia acts by rendering the circuit refractory; however, it is the least effective method of pacing for tachycardia

B – **T** this method saturates the re-entrant circuit and is effective in atrial flutter and junctional arrhythmias. It may accelerate ventricular tachycardia or convert it to fibrillation

C – **F** but it is a technique best left to experts as it requires specialist equipment to administer very precisely timed premature stimuli

D – **T** pacing at a rate faster than the sinus rate may reduce the tendency for recurrence once the arrhythmia has been terminated

E – **T** junctional tachycardias terminated by either; atrial arrhythmias are best terminated by atrial pacing

13. A – **F** some patients spontaneously vomit and this action terminates a junctional tachycardia. Ipecachuana can be given to patients in whom vomiting is known to be effective

B – **F** it is unnecessary for the patient to actually immerse the head in water. This manoeuvre is highly effective in children and only requires facial wetting

C – **T** this technique is not advisable as it is uncomfortable for the patient, is ineffective, and seldom works if other methods have failed

D – **T** the patient should be supine, carotid bruits should not be present and massage should be rotary or longitudinal

E – **T** terminating about 50% of junctional arrhythmias. The patient should blow a sphygmomanometer to about 40–60 mm mercury and hold this for 15 sec. The arrhythmia usually terminates during the relaxation after this

ARTERIAL PULSE

14. A – **F** febrile states such as typhoid cause intense vasodilatation and a dicrotic pulse, even in the presence of a normal aortic valve

B – **F** this type of pulse is found in mitral regurgitation and ventricular septal defect, due to 'ventricular runoff'

C – **F** although associated with aortic regurgitation, this abnormality may also be found in conditions of arterio-venous fistula, either natural or man-made, and in severe anaemia and thyrotoxicosis

D – **T** the paradoxical pulse, which is a rise in pulse pressure on *expiration* is a feature of pericardial tamponade or acute, severe asthma

E – **T** pulsus alternans is found with varying cardiac outputs in heart failure. Pulsus bisferiens is the abnormal notched pulse that represents a mixed aortic valve problem

ATRIAL FIBRILLATION

15. A – **F** the risk of stroke is 5% a year
B – **T** to about 1.5% a year
C – **F** patients aged under 60 with chronic or paroxysmal atrial fibrillation and no underlying heart disease have a very low incidence of these complications
D – **T** the risk of important bleeding is about 0.5% a year
E – **T** but not to the same extent as warfarin (SPAF study. Circulation. 1991;84:527)

16. A – **T** aspirin at this dose is of no proven benefit (AFASAK study. Lancet. 1989;i:175)
B – **F** aspirin reduces the relative risk by 42%: from 6.3% on placebo to 3.6% (SPAF study. Circulation. 1991;84:527)
C – **F** although beneficial, no direct comparison is possible with warfarin as yet
D – **T**
E – **F** there was no significant increase in serious haemorrhagic events with aspirin

ATRIAL NATRIURETIC FACTOR

17. A – **F** ANF is secreted mainly by the left atrial appendage in a healthy heart, but also by the left ventricle in heart failure
B – **T** an increase in ANF secretion results from an increased filling pressure in either ventricle
C – **T** ANF production is increased if the Na intake goes up and falls if Na intake is reduced. This mechanism helps to maintain the constancy of the blood volume, i.e. the constancy of the 'milieu interne' (Claude Bernard)
D – **F** as effective diuretic treatment reduces the level of Na in the blood, the ANF level will fall
E – **T** ANF increases blood pressure by stimulating the activity of plasma renin

AUSCULTATION OF THE HEART

18. A – **T** the third heart sound represents rapid filling of the left ventricle in early diastole

B – **T** as the fourth sound is caused by atrial systole at the end of diastole, it will disappear in atrial fibrillation

C – **T** a gallop rhythm is not uncommon in patients up to the age of 30 years, without indicating the presence of cardiac disease

D – **F** a fourth sound is present and is due to altered compliance of the left ventricle and is often heard in any condition causing an increase in end diastolic pressure, e.g. HOCM, aortic stenosis, hypertension. Its clinical significance is that it indicates left ventricular strain

E – **T** may occur normally in young healthy adults and is thought to be due to sudden limitation of filling of the left ventricle. In older patients it is always abnormal and usually indicates failure of one or other ventricle

19. A – **T** normally the aortic valve closes first and the later closure of the pulmonary valve is the cause of a splitting of the second sound

B – **F** it is in pulmonary stenosis that they are split and the pulmonary component of the second sound is very faint

C – **T** the second sound will be fixed and split. The lack of splitting of the second sound may suggest Fallot's tetralogy, severe stenosis of the pulmonary or aortic valves, pulmonary atresia, a large VSD or hypertension

D – **F** it may represent a patent ductus: the continuous systolic and diastolic murmur, heard at the left sternal edge frequently obscures the second heart sound

E – **T** in transposition, the aortic second sound is both loud and palpable at the upper sternum, being generated from the anteriorly placed aorta – the pulmonary second sound is often inaudible due to its usual softness and its posterior placement

β-BLOCKERS

20. A – **T** although non-selective β-blockers do reduce the awareness of hypoglycaemia, selective agents are less likely to do so and may be given; β-blockers may increase the blood sugar levels by up to 1.5 mmol/L and doses require adjustment accordingly

B – **T** non-selective β-blockers without intrinsic sympathomimetic activity (e.g. propranolol, sotalol, nadolol) should be avoided but β-blockers with high ISA, e.g. pindolol, or cardioselective agents may be given

C – **F** agents with low hepatic clearance, such as atenolol, nadolol, sotalol and pindolol, can safely be used. If plasma protein levels are reduced, then β-blockers that are highly protein bound, such as propranolol or pindolol should be avoided

D – **F** β-blockers with a reasonable indication may be continued throughout the perioperative period. If the indication is trivial, they should be stopped 48 hours before surgery, as they may result in excessive bradycardia, heart failure, and other effects possibly enhanced by an interaction with anaesthetic agents

E – **F** although severe asthma is an absolute contraindication, patients with mild bronchospasm or chronic airways obstruction may receive cardioselective agents with the co-prescription of β_2 stimulants

21. A – **F** if the angina is due to coronary spasm the β-blockers may enhance that artery spasm, due to unopposed α-receptor activity; β-blockers should therefore be avoided in Prinzmetal's variant angina, the basis of which is severe coronary spasm

B – **F** when combined with nifedipine in the treatment of angina, or hypertension, they reduce the resultant tachycardia. However, they should only be combined with verapamil cautiously because of potential AV block

C – **T** β-blockers are less effective in the elderly and these patients are more prone to side-effects. These patients are better started on a mild diuretic or a vasodilator

D – **T** the young non-smoking white male patient, with co-existent angina is the best responder to β-blockers: black patients respond better to vasodilators or the combined α- and β-blocker, labetalol.

E – **F** the ideal β-blocker would be long acting, cardioselective, effective in the standard dose, have a simple metabolic pathway (no liver metabolism, little protein binding, lipid insoluble and no active metabolites) and would be vasodilatory and either have ISA or be α-blocking. Atenolol meets nearly all those ideals, other than lack of intrinsic sympathomimetic activity

22. A – **T** it has been found in clinical studies that propranolol has to be withdrawn in about 10% of patients and atenolol in 2%. Both can cause fatigue, cold extremeties and worsening claudication, dreams and bronchospasm

B – **T** this side-effect is surprisingly rare if the correct contraindications (patients known to have suffered cardiac failure or to have poor cardiac function) are adhered to and proper patient selection occurs

C – **F** it has occasionally been found that when used as mono-therapy, hypertension may be aggravated. However, this is related to increased fluid retention in patients with low renin levels

D – **F** pindolol causes less fall in cardiac output because of its high intrinsic sympathomimetic activity. Labetalol, because of its α-blocking activity also causes less bradycardia and fall in cardiac output

E – **F** propranolol causes vidid dreams by this mechanism but dreams in patients on pindolol are thought to be caused by the insomnia resulting from the relatively high sympathetic tone at night which results from its high intrinsic sympathomimetic activity

23. A – **T** the α-mediated rebound hypertension caused by clonidine withdrawal will be exacerbated by the presence of a β-blocker

B – **F** reserpine acts by causing a depletion of catecholamines, so interfering with the sympathomimetic properties of the β-blocker, which may thus have reduced effects

C – **F** cimetidine reduces hepatic blood flow so blood levels of propranolol, which is metabolised in the liver, will be increased. In patients on cimetidine, it may be better to use β-blockers which are not metabolised in the liver, such as atenolol, sotalol and nadolol

D – **T** by combining a β-blocker with nifedipine, the reflex tachycardia induced by the fall in blood pressure is reduced by the β-blocker, thus enhancing the hypotensive effect of the nifedipine

E – **T** the fluid retention caused by the NSAIDs counteracts the hypotensive effects of the β-blocker

24. A – **F** none of the currently available calcium antagonists is contraindicated in asthma – all β-blockers require caution and some (those which are not cardioselective) are contraindicated

B – **F** the calcium-channel blockers have no such effect but the β-blockers may alter the ratio of high-density to low-density lipoproteins in an unfavourable way (the HDL cholesterol is reduced by unclear mechanisms and this is theoretically undesirable). The calcium antagonists have no such effect

C – **T** verapamil and diltiazem are negatively-inotropic and relatively contraindicated in cardiac failure but nicardipine and amlodipine may be given as they do not significantly depress myocardial contractility

D – **F** verapamil and diltiazem, together with β-blockers, should not be used in patients with digitalis toxicity, and they should also be used with care in patients on digoxin, even if toxicity is not evident. Nifedipine can also be used in combination with digitalis without toxicity

E – **F** nifedipine should be avoided in cardiomyopathy, as its vasodilator properties may increase the gradient across the obstruction. The other calcium antagonists and the β-blockers are not thought to do this

25. A – **F** sotalol alone prolongs the action potential. All the β-blockers limit the production of tissue cyclic AMP and this gives them their anti-arrhythmic activity

B – **F** stimulation of the central nervous system at night, when sympathetic tone is low, may result in poor sleep

C – **T** atenolol > metoprolol > acebutalol in selectivity of cardiac activity, but all β-blockers cause some degree of bronchospasm, usually at higher doses, and all should be avoided or used with caution in patients with chronic obstructive lung disease or asthma

D – **T** although high ISA may diminish the bronchospasm induced by β-blockade, it will also lessen the response of the airways to β-agonist inhalers – thus a cardioselective β-blocker would be the β-blocker of choice in patients with airway obstruction

E – **T** labetalol also causes less bronchospasm, but the two major consequences are postural hypotension in high doses, and retrograde ejaculation in men due to relaxation of the bladder neck sphincter

CARDIAC AND BRONCHIAL ASTHMA

26. A – **F** diffuse wheezing can occur in both conditions. In BA the wheezing tends to be more high-pitched and musical

B – **T** the sweating skin is a distinctive feature of LVF and is due to compensatory sympathetic overactivity

C – **T** a gallop rhythm is very frequent in LVF, and if due to a fourth heart sound is virtually diagnostic. A gallop rhythm is rare in BA unless it is associated with long-standing chronic obstructive lung disease and cor pulmonale

D – **F** Curschmann's sign is coughing up spirals of thick stringy mucus, and occurs in bronchial asthma

E – **T** cyanosis is common in LVF due to decreased cutaneous blood flow and arterial desaturation due to the pulmonary congestion. While arterial hypoxaemia is present in BA it is not usually of sufficient degree to cause cyanosis

CARDIAC ARRHYTHMIAS

27. A – **T** there is no warning before the loss of consciousness and this helps differentiate it from epilepsy

B – **F** but a tonic–clonic seizure may result from the cerebral hypoxia caused by asystole

C – **F** the collapse is associated with pallor due to arrested circulation but the recovery is often heralded by a profound flushing as the circulation returns and this is a characteristic feature noted by witnesses

D – **F** and rapid return of consciousness helps to differentiate a Stoke–Adams attack from an epileptic seizure

E – **F** the episode of loss of consciousness is usually very transient and recovery is rapid

CARDIAC DRUGS

28. A – **T** nitroprusside is converted to thiocyanate and high levels of this inhibit the thyroid gland, causing a hypothyroid state

B – **F** the conversion of the metabolites of the nitroprusside to cyanocobalamins enhances excretion and reduces toxic side-effects. Thus concurrent hydroxycobalamin should be administered

C – **F** it inhibits cytochrome oxidase in the liver, into which it freely diffuses, and causes hypoxic damage to hepatocytes

D – **T** 90% of the free cyanide is erythrocyte bound and due to cytochrome oxidase inhibition, interferes with aerobic metabolism

E – **T** the metabolites of nitroprusside are renally excreted and have a long half-life of about 7 days

CARDIAC GLYCOSIDES

29. A – **T** although ouabain acts rapidly after intravenous therapy (within 1 hour), it is not used orally, and if i.v. administration is effective, a switch to oral digoxin should be made subsequently

B – **T** the half-life of digitoxin is between 4 and 6 days, although its hepatic metabolism and gut excretion make it useful in patients with renal failure requiring glycosides

C – **T** it has similar actions and indications to digoxin but causes less gastrointestinal upset – it is rarely used except when patients are intolerant of other glycosides

D – **F** its maximum benefit is 2–3 hours after it has been given, and oral digoxin, which is rapidly absorbed, is likely to be just as effective – and cheaper

E – **T** digoxin is the preferred glycoside, and it has a half-life of 1–2 days, which is why it can be administered as a once daily treatment

CARDIAC SURGERY

30. A – **T** both these mechanical valves have a low incidence of mechanical failure and are reliable and long lasting

B – **F** most valves have a high incidence of thromboembolism if not anticoagulated – and many whether warfarinised or not, but in general all valves other than the tissue valves should receive lifelong anticoagulation

C – **T** tissue degeneration is likely to occur from 7 years after implantation. Destruction is rapid once it has presented and replacement should be carried out as a matter of urgency

D – **F** prosthetic endocarditis is not related to the valve position and is more common in patients whose valve was replaced for bacterial endocarditis than for rheumatic or ischaemic disease

E – **F** it is rare, even in a mechanical valve if functioning normally so the presence of haemolysis should alert the clinician to the possibility of a paraprosthetic leak

CARDIAC THERAPY

31. A – **T** particularly with captopril to reduce the first-dose hypotensive effect. Advise patient to take the first dose last thing at night or to stay in bed for some hours after taking the tablet

B – **F** but frequently (one or two weekly) especially in patients with heart failure and renal impairment, as significant potassium retention may occur, particularly in the first few days

C – **F** this is not necessary unless there is a reason to suspect renal artery disease (e.g. young patient with severe hypertension resistant to usual therapy). ACE inhibitors may cause renal failure in patients with unexpected renal artery stenosis – especially if unilateral

D – **F** but probably advisable for patients requiring ACE inhibitors for heart failure rather than hypertension because the former are more likely to be on diuretics and be prone to the adverse effects on renal function and serum potassium levels

E – **T** the dose of loop diuretics (e.g. frusemide and bumetanide) should be at least halved a day before the introduction of ACE inhibitors, to improve the vascular 'state' and so avoid postural hypotension. Any potassium-sparing diuretic should be withdrawn to prevent severe hyperkalaemia

CARDIAC TRANSPLANTATION

32. A – **T** even with currently used immunosuppressives, rejection occurs at least once in >90% recipients. Early signs of a rejection include the development of 3rd and 4th heart sounds and diminution of QRS voltages on the ECG

B – **F** a pulmonary vascular resistance of >8 Wood units is a contraindication to transplant unless it is combined with a lung transplant, because this would rapidly cause right heart failure in the donor heart

C – **F** azathioprine and corticosteroids, the former at the highest level compatible with an adequate white cell and platelet count; the latter at the lowest dose necessary to prevent rejection

D – F nearly all patients sustain at least one infective episode. The majority are bacterial infections of the lung and usually correspond to high levels of immunosuppression, being commonest in the first three months after surgery

E – T accelerated atherosclerosis in the donor heart is a serious case of late morbidity and mortality and may be reduced by low lipid diet, exercise and antiplatelet therapy

CARDIAC TRAUMA

33. A – T angina may occur early after the injury, even in the absence of coronary disease on angiography. The cause of this post-traumatic angina is unknown

B – T pericardial injury from blunt trauma is common. On autopsy, 50% of cases have evidence of pericardial damage following non-penetrating injuries to the heart

C – T this is usually due to rupture of the chordae tendinae and papillary muscle, rather than to damage to the valve itself

D – F the commonest cause of death is rupture of the heart

E – F any increase in cardiac enzymes might well be due to damage to the non-cardiac structures. The best simple diagnostic test is the ECG which often shows evidence of pericarditis when cardiac damage has occurred from non-penetrating injury

CHOLESTEROL AND HEART DISEASE

34. A – F lowering the blood cholesterol does not increase deaths from myocardial infarction but it can lead to an increased mortality from non-cardiac causes

B – T the initial trials with clofibrate in 1978 highlighted an increased death rate from bowel cancer. This finding has been somewhat controversial, and subsequent trials have both supported and denied the association. A definitive answer to this question is probably still to come

C – **T** the increased mortality has been found at least in part to be due to an increase in violent death, including suicide

D – **T** it has been suggested that low blood cholesterol levels result in neurochemical changes in the brain leading to alteration of the cell membranes. It is possible that this cellular change can affect the patient's behaviour

E – **F** the adverse mortality findings in different trials have not been found to depend on the type of drug used. It appears to be the actual lowering of the level of blood cholesterol which is the relevant factor

CHRONIC CONSTRICTIVE PERICARDITIS

35. A – **T** in developed nations most cases are of unknown aetiology, except in children where TB is still an important cause. It is also important in developing countries

B – **F** pulsus paradoxus is rarely present because there are no major inspiratory swings of right ventricular filling pressure

C – **F** left ventricular function is normal in both conditions

D – **T** complete resection of the pericardium is the best treatment – it carries a 5-year survival rate of 85%

E – **F** it is 3 times as common in men as in women

CLINICAL EXAMINATION

36. A – **F** the normal apex beat should be palpable but should not raise the examining finger

B – **F** the apex will be thrusting in hypertension, aortic stenosis and hypertrophic cardiomyopathy

C – **T** if it is hyperdynamic and displaced, consider regurgitation of mitral or aortic valves or a VSD: the apex is diffuse in cardiac failure

D – **F** but it may not be palpable for many reasons, e.g. obesity, lung disease – consider dextrocardia in a patient who appears slim and normal but in whom the apex cannot be palpated

E – T a double impulse may also be apparent in cases of HCM and mitral valve prolapse

CONGENITAL HEART BLOCK

37. A – **T** in general the prognosis is worse in familial cases especially if associated with wide QRS complexes. In uncomplicated non-familial cases the prognosis is likely to be good, with 95% surviving for at least 20 years

B – **T** the haemodynamic response to exercise and other stresses is reasonably normal in uncomplicated cases (absence of other cardiac malformations) because there is usually a stable accelerated junctional pacemaker under autonomic control, allowing some increase in heart rate during exercise

C – **F** congenital CHB can be associated with malignant ventricular tachy-arrhythmias, therefore it is desirable to carry out exercise testing and/or Holter monitoring to decide whether anti-arrhythmic drugs or pacing is indicated

D – **T** it may follow SLE or other connective tissue disease in the mother

E – **F** usually pregnancy is uneventful in these women, though Stokes–Adams attacks may occur soon after delivery and temporary pacing may be desirable in these women if they have marked bradycardia

38. A – **F** in most cases the heart is completely normal, and the cause of the CHB is unknown. Rarely, the condition may be associated with corrected transposition of the great arteries

B – **T** systemic lupus erythematosus in the mother can cause CHB in the baby, probably by the passage of immune complexes through the placenta

C – **T** provided the child survives infancy the prognosis is good and the child usually remains asymptomatic until adolescence. The presence of an associated cardiovascular abnormality considerably reduces the chance of survival. A 20-year survival of 95% has been reported in the absence of any other cardiac abnormality

D – **F** pregnancy is usually uneventful. Rarely, Stokes–Adams attacks may occur, and these can be treated easily with a pacemaker

E – **F** congenital CHB occurs with equal frequency in males and females

CONGENITAL HEART DISEASE

39. A – **T**

B – **T** an isolated VSD affects about 2 in every 1000 live births

C – **F** spontaneous closure occurs in 30–50% of patients

D – **F** a VSD will cause this and it is the commonest cause of 'hyperkinetic' pulmonary hypertension, which will be evidenced by a chest X-ray showing pulmonary plethora and an enlarged pulmonary artery

E – **F** less than 10% of patients with VSD also have a patent duct

CORONARY ARTERY DISEASE

40. A – **T** there is a variable heart rate response. Inferior ischaemia is associated with a slight bradycardia whereas anterior ischaemia causes a tachycardia

B – **T** the LVEDP rises uniformly as the ischaemia persists, although systemic BP initially falls then rises in response to the continued pain

C – **T** narrowing of 25–30% is frequently seen in such patients. It is believed that coronary artery spasm only rarely occurs in normal coronary arteries

D – **F** the aetiology is more complex and it is not known what is the cause. Active influences include endogenous vasoconstrictors and endothelial damage causing loss of endothelium-dependent vasodilator substances. These factors may influence the activation of vascular smooth muscle

E – **T** there is evidence that myocardial oxygen demand does not change, but 'simply' is reduced: ST segment elevation occurs in about 35% of patients during chest pain and ergometrine induces spasm in 15–20% of patients

DIGOXIN

41. A – **T** 75% is absorbed rapidly and the rest is inactivated by organisms in the lower intestine prior to excretion

B – **T** digoxin is lipid soluble and so crosses the blood–brain barrier, although this is thought to be of little clinical significance

C – **T** digoxin does not bind to plasma proteins and has a half-life of about 36 hours

D – **F** most of the circulating digoxin is excreted unchanged by the kidneys and so dosage restriction is necessary in patients with renal impairment

E – **F** in hyperthyroidism, malabsorption syndromes, and drugs which interfere with absorption (such as cholestyramine, neomycin, rifampicin) may all be associated with low serum levels of digoxin: the mechanism for this is unknown

DISSECTION OF THE AORTA

42. A – **T** the mortality is about 30% within the first two days

B – **T** dissection with pericardial tamponade is the commonest mode of death in these patients

C – **F** the usual target is a systolic pressure of 100 mm or less for the younger patient and 120 mm for the elderly, previously hypertensive patient. This level of pressure can be induced with a labetalol infusion at a rate of 125 μg to 2 mg/minute

D – **F** if no complications occur, as is frequent with a posterior dissection. If complications such as loss of pulses, pericardial rupture or aortic regurgitation occur, surgery is a priority

E – **T** an ostial stenosis of the right coronary artery may be a complication of a proximal aortic dissection and may itself require treatment

DRIVING REGULATIONS AND CARDIOVASCULAR DISEASE

43. A – **T**
B – **F** unless the root is >5 cm – whatever the cause
C – **F** if, 3 months later, the patient is angina free and can complete a negative exercise test
D – **T** an aneurysm of >4 cm combined with evidence of cardiac ischaemia
E – **F** unless co-existent angina also affects the patient

44. A – **F** as long as the blood pressure is <180/100
B – **T** any casual reading of >200/110 will bar the patient from holding such a licence
C – **F** as long as the medication is digoxin, verapamil or a β-blocker
D – **F** as long as the patient is asymptomatic and attending a pacemaker clinic annually
E – **T**

45. A – **F** unnecessary if the exercise test at >3 months post-infarction is normal
B – **F** if the ejection fraction is found to be less than 40% the licence will not be returned
C – **F** if single vessel disease does not involve the left main stem or the LAD proximal to the first septal or diagonal vessel, the licence may be returned
D – **T** significant disease of 2 or more major coronary arteries is not permissible for such a licence
E – **F** (see answer to C above)

46. A – **F** the licence must be surrendered for at least 3 months but may be reinstated if he can complete at least 3 stages of a Bruce treadmill protocol successfully
B – **F** see answer to A above
C – **F** he has to complete 3 stages only, without significant cardiac symptoms, serious arrhythmias and no pathological ST depression
D – **T** see answer to C above
E – **F** an angiogram is unnecessary if a treadmill test is completed and the patient is free of angina

DRUG THERAPY IN HEART DISEASE

47. A – **T** nitrates are predominantly venous vasodilators and improve cardiac failure by reducing the venous return to the heart
B – **T** nitroprusside is equally effective for arterial and venous vasodilatation. It is rapidly active, has a short half-life and may quickly be titrated against response. It is also potentially toxic and should be infused for relatively short periods by a large central vein
C – **T** infusions of this sympathomimetic may cause hypokalaemia and increase the tendency towards arrhythmias
D – **T** an infusion of nitroprusside causes anaerobic metabolism and the subsequent build-up of lactate in the arteries causes a metabolic acidosis
E – **F** hydralazine is predominantly an arterial dilator and causes a reduction in blood pressure, a fall in afterload and a reflex tachycardia

EBSTEIN'S ANOMALY

48. A – **F** the right ventricular muscle and chordae tendinae are often highly malformed leading to considerable variation in the manner of attachment of the tricuspid valve to the right ventricular wall
B – **F** it is pulmonary atresia which may accompany Ebstein's

anomaly in infants

C – **T** the first heart sound is loud and split and the second heart sound is widely and persistently split. Third and fourth heart sounds are not usually heard in infants, but may be present in older patients

D – **F** there is a very distinctive ECG with giant peaked P waves, a prolonged P–Q interval and frequently right bundle branch block

E – **T** the diagnostic feature in cardiac catheterisation is on withdrawing the catheter from the right ventricle to the right atrium – in the proximal area of the right ventricle the ECG will be right ventricular but the pressure curve is atrial in contour

ECG

49. A – **T** it occurs in WPW syndrome, type A

B – **F** a dominant R in V1 occurs in true posterior infarction only, with accompanying changes in lead III but not in aVF. A postero-inferior infarction has changes of infarction in III aVF and often V5 and V6

C – **F** although V1 shows a conduction defect pattern, the R wave is minimal

D – **T** left posterior hemiblock with or without myocardial infarction produces a large R in V1

E – **F** hyperkalaemia produces peaked T waves not R waves

50. A – **T** left axis deviation is said to occur when the cardiac axis is between −30 and −90 degrees. If the axis is between −90 and 180 degrees, extreme left axis deviation is present

B – **F** a secundum ASD typically causes a right axis shift on the ECG because of the right ventricular hypertrophy resulting from left-to-right shunting of blood

C – **T** the ostium primum ASD is associated with left axis deviation because of mitral valve involvement and the associated mitral incompetence leading to left ventricular hypertrophy

D – **T** posterior hemi-block is shown as right bundle branch block

E – **T** severe pulmonary stenosis may result in deviation of the axis to the right due to marked right ventricular hypertrophy

FIBRINOLYTIC THERAPY

51. A – **T** compared TPA 100 mg/3 hours to placebo in 5011 patients with a history suggestive of MI within 5 hours of onset of main symptoms (ECG changes were not mandatory)

B – **F** all patients had a heparin bolus at the time of administration of TPA and then an infusion of heparin for 24 hours. Aspirin was not given

C – **T** the 1 month mortality was reduced by 26%, from 9.8% to 7.2%

D – **T** benefit with TPA was confined to patients who had ECG evidence of myocardial infarction

E – **T** although overall incidence of stroke was similar in both groups of patients, haemorrhagic stroke was more common in the TPA group and thrombotic stroke more frequent in placebo patients

Wilcox RG (for ASSET Study Group). Trial of tissue plasminogen activator for mortality reduction in acute myocardial infarction (ASSET). Lancet. 1988;2:525–30.

52. A – **F** after TPA it does enhance the action of the drug and reduce rethrombosis but after the non-fibrin-specific agents (streptokinase and APSAC), which themselves produce a hypocoagulable state, it is not essential

B – **F** platelet activation is reduced and because of this, anticoagulants are less effective than anti-platelet agents in preventing thrombosis in arterial vessels

C – **F** the high rates of rethrombosis after fibrinolytic therapy are not reduced by the co-administration of heparin, which itself augments the platelet activation of lytic therapy

D – **T** the high-molecular-weight heparins bind to platelets, causing activation and subsequent aggregation, thrombosis and thrombocytopenia

E – **F** heparin-activated antithrombin III blocks the action of thrombin in the blood but cannot inhibit fibrin formed on platelet surfaces

HEART MURMURS

53. A – **T** they are common in children and young adults

B – **T** a diastolic heart murmur must never be considered innocent and unimportant

C – **F** added sounds, such as an ejection click, do not occur with entirely innocent murmurs

D – **T** an innocent murmur is usually best heard down the left edge of the sternum but may be heard elsewhere

E – **T** it is sensible to do a chest X-ray, ECG and echo to confirm the benign nature of the murmur before dismissing it

HYPERTENSION

54. 1 – C
2 – A
3 – B
4 – B, D
5 – A, B

55. 1 – C
2 – D
3 – A
4 – E
5 – B

56. A – **F** patient should be seated
B – **F** measure pressure to the nearest 2 mmHg mercury
C – **F** take 2 measurements at each of the 4 visits (mean of 8 readings) before labelling a patient as hypertensive
D – **T** the elderly and diabetics commonly have postural hypotension
E – **T** in milder hypertensives without end-organ damage and in the older patient

57. A – **F** systolics of >160 mmHg should be treated
B – **T** as long as systolic pressure is <161 mmHg
C – **T** but if they are already on treatment, this should be continued
D – **F** isolated systolic pressures of >160 mmHg should be treated regardless of diastolic pressure
E – **T** as aggressive reduction of diastolic pressure may increase coronary risk

INFECTIVE ENDOCARDITIS

58. A – **T** more than half the cases are on abnormal valves
B – **F** *Strep. viridans* is responsible for about 75% of infections in non-geriatric medical patients, but this falls to 50% with an increase in *Strep. faecalis* and *Staph. epidermidis*, and Gram-negative organisms from the bowel in elderly patients
C – **F** multiple infection should be suspected if the initial response is followed by a relapse and a different organism is found in the blood culture
D – **T** a single antibiotic, even if broad-spectrum should not be the initial choice: two antibiotics should be used for a synergistic effect and to reduce the development of resistant organisms. Benzyl penicillin combined with gentamicin is the usual starting combination unless staphylococcal infection is suspected, when flucloxacillin should be used as well
E – **T** although 6 weeks treatment should be the general rule and, in the absence of complications, patients should

usually have been afebrile for 14 days before treatment is discontinued. The treatment does not need to be by the intravenous route in all cases. Straightforward *Strep. viridans* infections can usually be treated with 14 days intravenous penicillin and gentamicin, then a further two weeks of oral amoxicillin. *Strep. faecalis* should always be treated for 6 weeks with parenteral penicillin and gentamicin.

INOTROPIC SYMPATHOMIMETIC MEDICATION

59. A – **F** it causes vasoconstriction which is mediated through α-receptors in the vessel walls

B – **T** intravenous isoprenaline causes a tachycardia due to stimulation of the β_1-receptors in the wall of the ventricle

C – **T** noradrenaline is released from myocardial cells in response to stimulation by dopamine

D – **F** it is dobutamine that has this action which is mediated through the stimulation of β_2-receptors in the walls of peripheral vessels

E – **F** although both β_1- and β_2-receptors are affected, there is only a weak β_2-stimulating effect and most actions are β_1-mediated

INSULIN AND HEART DISEASE

60. A – **T** hyperinsulinaemia is associated with an increased risk of atherosclerosis, though this is more marked in European than black people. It may be that it is not the hyperinsulinaemia itself which is the relevant risk factor but the accompanying insulin resistance leading to hypertriglyceridaemia

B – **T** insulin stimulates vascular smooth muscle proliferation and lipid deposition

C – **F** hyperinsulinaemia is associated with hypertension, and this may well contribute to the increased risk of atherosclerosis

D – **F** the University Group Diabetes Programme did not show any adverse effects of insulin treatment on cardiovascular complications [1]

E – **F** although nicotinic acid causes hyperinsulinaemia and insulin resistance, it actually decreased cardiovascular mortality in men with coronary artery disease [2]

[1] The UGDP. Effects of hypoglycaemic agents on the vascular complications in patients with adult onset diabetes. Diabetes. 1982;(suppl 5):1–77.

[2] Canner PL, Berge JD, Wenger NK et al. 15 year mortality in coronary drug project patients. Long term benefits with niacin. J Am Coll Cardiol. 1986;8:1245–55.

MARFAN SYNDROME

61. A – **F** males predominate; the range is from 2:1 up to 8:1 in different series

B – **T** though these are very much in a minority. Cardiac complications occur in at least 60% of patients

C – **F** although it is true that the predominant cardiac abnormality in Marfan syndrome is a dilatation of the aortic ring, the sinuses of Valsalva and the ascending aorta, the mitral valve can also be involved in myxomatous degeneration and prolapse

D – **T** blue sclerae may occur in Marfan syndrome. The other 2 conditions in which blue sclerae occur are Ehlers–Danlos syndrome and osteogenesis imperfecta

E – **T** as aortic dissection is a potentially fatal complication in Marfan syndrome, β-blocking drugs have been used on the basis of a resultant reduction in the force of cardiac contraction on the already damaged aortic wall

MATERNAL MORTALITY DUE TO HEART DISEASE IN PREGNANCY

62. A – **F** it is the third commonest. Hypertension and thrombo-embolism are the commonest

B – **F** the incidence of acquired heart disease has halved, and that of congenital heart disease has doubled

C – **F** the same report indicated that the main cause was coronary disease

D – **T** a third of patients with puerperal cardiomyopathy will die in spite of modern drug treatment. In these patients the only treatment which can improve survival is cardiac transplantation

E – **F** anticoagulants are the treatment of choice antenatally to avoid the serious risk of pulmonary embolism

METABOLIC HEART DISEASE

63. A – **F** myocardial damage is very rare in phaeochromocytoma. On the other hand, heart failure is common in untreated patients because of the strain of the increased metabolic demands

B – **T** a short P–R interval is common in glycogen storage disease and may precipitate WPW syndrome

C – **T** when cardiac involvement occurs it affects the right ventricle rather than the left

D – **T** 15% of patients have cardiac involvement in haemachromatosis. Since the diabetes is usually controllable with insulin, heart failure is the commonest cause of death, especially if extensive cardiac fibrosis is present

E – **F** the infant may be born with either diffuse hyperplasia or hypertrophy, or changes localised to the left ventricle and septum, like HOCM. The cardiac involvement is reversible within 12 months in some infants

MITRAL REGURGITATION

64. A – **F** it may be loudest at the left sternal edge if the jet is directed at the anterior wall of the left atrium

B – **T** anterior chordal rupture leads to a loud posterior murmur: posterior chordal rupture causes the murmur to be heard best at the left sternal edge

C – **T** mitral regurgitation is best seen by screening in the 30 degree right anterior oblique position

D – **F** the size of the left atrium is also related to the severity of the regurgitation. If the LA is greatly enlarged, it will 'absorb' some of the regurgitant pressure and so reduce the 'v' wave seen at catheterisation: this occurs in chronic, as opposed to acute, mitral regurgitation

E – **F** there is 60% survival at 5 years after diagnosis on medical treatment alone

MITRAL STENOSIS

65. A – **T** it may co-exist with an atrial septal defect in the inherited Lutembacher syndrome: which may be confused with rheumatic mitral stenosis and a patent foramen ovale

B – **T** the usual infecting organism is of the group A streptococcal family (usually type 12) and the antigen antibody reaction caused damages the valve

C – **T** the best test for diagnosis and differentiation is echocardiography: the catheter used for angiocardiography may cause parts of the myxoma to become detached and to embolise

D – **T** this is due to reduced cardiac output in patients with moderate or severe stenosis. On exertion, if the cardiac output is doubled, the gradient across the valve is quadrupled and this increases the pulmonary capillary wedge pressure and restricts exertion. The presence of atrial fibrillation further reduces cardiac output

E – **T** the enlargement of the left atrium will also compress other structures such as the recurrent laryngeal nerve – resulting in hoarseness (Ortner syndrome); and the left main bronchus (left lung collapse)

66. A – **F** the more stenosed the mitral valve, the softer is the first sound. A loud first sound is due to a 'still mobile' mitral valve being 'slammed' shut at the onset of ventricular systole

B – **F** the closer the opening snap is to the aortic 2nd sound, the tighter the stenosis. This is because the left atrial pressure increases progressively with the severity of the mitral valve stenosis, and the higher the pressure, the earlier the mitral valve will open in diastole

C – **T** the more severe the stenosis, the longer the duration of diastolic flow and the murmur

D – **T** if mitral regurgitation coexists and predominates, a third heart sound will often be audible

E – **F** chronic lung disease is common and this is thought to be due to oedematous bronchial mucosa which is prone to infection

MITRAL VALVE SYNDROME

67. A – **T** a floppy mitral valve is thought to be present in about 5% of the normal population

B – **F** due to progressive stretching of the leaflets and weakening caused by deposition of acid mucopolysaccharides in the zona spongiosa – both leaflets are usually affected

C – **T** and the impulse is thought to be caused by an increase in the tension of the chordae which occurs in the middle of systole

D – **F** a mid-systolic click may be heard which occurs after the carotid upstroke of the pulse which helps differentiate it from a similar but earlier sound in aortic stenosis

E – **T** the murmurs of MVP and HOCM are both accentuated after amyl nitrate – and HOCM does not have a midsystolic click and therefore may be differentiated from MVP

MYOCARDIAL INFARCTION

68. A – **T** it is believed to be a sign of ischaemia in other areas, rather than merely a 'reflection' of the ST elevation in other areas

B – **F** patients demonstrating this on their acute ECG have greater enzyme rises and more in-hospital complications than patients without, suggesting it is related to the enormity of the infarction

C – **F** there is no convincing evidence that reciprocal change identifies diseased arteries remote from the site of the infarction, but merely indicates that other territories are involved

D – **T** although there may not be remote coronary artery disease, the ECG abnormalities may reflect a reduction in coronary flow, putting these patients at high risk of complications

E – **F** the area of reciprocal change is often the area where ST depression will occur on later exercise testing

69. 1 – A/iii recruiting 11,712 patients and assessing mortality at 21 days

2 – A/ii recruiting 1741 patients and assessing the 21-day mortality

3 – A/iv recruiting 17,187 patients and assessing mortality given for 5 weeks

4 – C/ii recruiting 1004 patients; mortality at 30 days

5 – B/i 5011 patients and 28-day mortality figures

70. A – **T** QRS changes may be found in patients who are later shown histologically to have had a subendocardial infarction and so should not be relied upon in the clinical diagnosis

B – **F** but early transmural infarction is often found in patients thought to have had a subendocardial infarction and subendocardial infarction is considered by many to be an intermediate state between crescendo angina and transmural myocardial infarction

C – **F** coronary vascular resistance rises with the high intramural tension in the subendocardium during systole. This virtually restricts perfusion of the subendocardium to diastole, and renders this zone vulnerable to ischaemic damage

D – **F** aortic stenosis is related to this type of infarction because of a combination of reduced coronary artery perfusion and increased left ventricular diastolic pressure, as a result of left ventricular hypertrophy both of which jeopardise the perfusion of the subendocardial zone

E – **T** cardiac massage can maintain effective cerebral circulation but coronary circulation is reduced to as little as 15% of the carotid circulation. This type of infarct should be sought after successful resuscitation

71. A – **T** about two-thirds of patients present with pain but they may have other presentations. In contrast, the vast majority of young patients with an infarction present because of pain

B – **T** only a small proportion of patients can be said to have a truly 'silent' infarct (2% in a recent study [1]). The mechanism is possibly a reduced sensitivity to pain in the older patients

C – **T** acute dyspnoea is the second most common presenting symptom of myocardial infarction in the elderly. The overwhelming dyspnoea may 'mask' the pain in the patient's perception and so present like a 'silent infarction'

D – **T** mortality rises with age but so does the difficulty in recognising the diagnosis. Accurate diagnosis is necessary before appropriate treatment so the possibility of an atypical presentation in an older patient is essential

E – **F** the fibrinolytic trials have shown that the benefits of treatment continue at all ages treated and as the elderly have a worse prognosis in view of their age, they are likely to have more to gain from such therapy

[1] Bayer AJ et al. J Am Geriatr Soc. 1986;34:263–6.

72. A – **T** 50% of patients dying after an inferior myocardial infarction are shown to have infarction of the right ventricle, and as much as 25% of the ventricular wall may be involved

B – **F** although this may be a manifestation of right ventricle infarction, it is neither sensitive nor specific. Even ST elevation in right precordial leads, although sensitive (>80%) has a specificity of between 40 and 90% so is unreliable

C – **T** severe RV dysfunction occurs in 10–20% of patients with RV infarction and has the characteristics of a right atrial pressure of >10 mm or a RA:wedge pressure ratio of >0.8

D – **F** it is fluids, rather than diuretics, that are required for the low output state that accompanies RV infarction. Always consider this possibility in a patient with inferior myocardial infarction followed by cardiogenic shock and be prepared to measure the left and right atrial pressures

E – **F** the typical findings of hypotension, oliguria, raised jugular venous pressure with Kusmaal's sign and clear lung fields differentiate it from pure LV failure

73. A – **T** typical pericardial pain occurs in about 28% of patients, a rub is detected in up to 20%, but a clinically significant pericardial effusion is uncommon

B – **T** an effusion, of itself, does not appear to increase the mortality. However, as its occurrence seems to be related to larger infarcts, anterior infarcts and left ventricular failure, it would appear to be a marker for those patients at higher risk of death

C – **T** although infrequently requiring drainage, an effusion may persist for six months after the infarction in a third of patients

D – **T** there is up to 50 ml fluid in the normal pericardial cavity and this may be misdiagnosed as an effusion. Pericardial fat, a coronary fistula and a pericardial tumour may also be indistinguishable from an effusion

E – **F** the fluid is thought to be the result of the oedema and inflammation that follows infarction and indicates that the healing process is active

74. A – **F** the cholesterol plaque ruptures first, platelets are deposited, the coagulation system is initiated and red blood cells and fibrin are deposited

B – **F** plaque fissuring is usually the initating event

C – **T** 20–50% of patients with non-Q wave infarction are shown to have total coronary artery occlusion

D – **F** studies have shown that prolonged infusions of TPA may result in progressive increase in arterial lumen and decrease in stenosis, although in most cases a significant (>70%) stenosis of the occluded coronary artery remains

E – **T** it has been shown that it is the exposure of the type I collagen fibres deep in the arterial media which stimulates platelet aggregation and thrombus formation. This is fixed deep in the artery wall and is likely to occlude the lumen

MYOCARDITIS

75. A – **F** a viral aetiology is suggested by a 4-fold rise in antibody titre in paired sera and a type-specific IgM with a titre of >1/32

B – **F** only 5% of patients suffering from a viral illness have cardiac involvement and histological evidence of viral myocarditis is present in 2–5% unselected autopsies and 17–21% of patients with unexpected cardiac death

C – **F** in males, the young and the pregnant, presenting as a subacute illness after a viral infection

D – **T** although the ECG is commonly abnormal, the changes are non-specific ST and T wave changes; arrhythmias and conduction disturbances may be the only sign of cardiac involvement

E – **T** steroids and immunosuppressives given in the early stages of the illness may actually increase cardiac damage, and most patients recover completely without such treatment

NITRATES

76. A – F the lack of first-pass metabolism of the mononitrates mean a more predictable response to therapy than the dinitrates, which undergo variable hepatic metabolism to mononitrate, which is the active component

B – T the constant, relatively high blood levels caused by wearing the patch are thought to be responsible for nitrate tolerance and reduced efficacy of the drug. A nitrate free interval, often during the night, is now recommended

C – F nitrates do reduce coronary spasm, but also cause dilatation of peripheral veins, reducing venous return and so limiting cardiac work – it is this effect which is most important in relieving angina

D – T their effect in reducing 'preload' benefits patients with cardiac failure by 'unloading' the circulation and so reducing cardiac work

E – F the hypotension caused when nitrates are combined with both β-blockers and calcium antagonists may make the patient feel worse, even if the angina is well controlled

77. A – T they are contraindicated in HOCM as they will cause vasodilatation of the major vessels which will increase the outflow obstruction and so reduce the cardiac output

B – F because they will reduce the diastolic filling of the already-compromised heart through reduction in the venous return, caused by peripheral vasodilatation

C – T nitrates are safe in anterior infarction, but may cause a reduction in the filling pressure and clinical deterioration in patients with acute inferior infarction and right ventricular involvement

D – T apart from amyl nitrite, there is no evidence that other nitrates cause a rise in intraocular pressure, and so they can be safely used in glaucoma

E – F sudden withdrawal of nitrates may lead to a clinical syndrome similar to that previously seen at the weekends in munition-factory workers during the last war (headaches each day of the week resolving at the weekend, when away from work for two days). Withdrawal should be gradual after long-term therapy as there have been reports of sudden death

78. A – F the combination of nitrates and hydralazine has been found to improve long-term survival in patients with chronic left ventricular failure

B – F nitrates are metabolized entirely in the liver

C – F nitrates are contraindicated in HOCM because they may reduce the left ventricular volume through peripheral venous pooling, and this will lead to a fall in cardiac output and a possible exacerbation of the angina

D – T again nitrates will reduce the diastolic filling of the heart due to peripheral venodilatation, and this will further impair the cardiac output

E – F there is no evidence that nitrates increase intraocular pressure, unlike amyl nitrite which is no longer used for treating angina

PAROXYSMAL ATRIAL FIBRILLATION (PAF)

79. A – F the Framingham study [1] showed that stroke incidence was 5.4% in sustained AF and only 1.3% in PAF

B – F digoxin is only of limited value in preventing attacks of PAF. Digoxin increases vagal tone and reduces the atrial refractory period, thus making the atrium more susceptible to attacks of fibrillation

C – T verapamil increases AV block and is therefore useful in controlling the ventricular rate in established AF. However, it has been found relatively ineffective in controlling recurrences in PAF. In addition, if given to a patient with WPW syndrome associated with the PAF, it can precipitate ventricular fibrillation

D – **F** simple ventricular pacing for PAF in sick-sinus syndrome leads to an increased incidence of permanent AF and heart failure [2]

E – **T** amiodarone is a very effective drug in PAF, especially in the elderly. Other drugs which may be of value include sotalol and propafenone

[1] Kannel WB, Abbott RD, Savage DD et al. Coronary heart disease and atrial fibrillation: the Framingham Study. Am Heart J. 1983;106:389–96.

[2] Hesselson AB, Parsonnet V, Bernstein AB et al. Deleterious effects of long-term single chamber ventricular pacing in sick-sinus-syndrome. J Am Coll Cardiol. 1992;19:1542–9.

PERCUTANEOUS, TRANSLUMINAL CORONARY ANGIOPLASTY

80. A – **T** restenosis may occur up to 6 months after the procedure; it is most likely in the first month after the angioplasty

B – **T** acute occlusion occurs in about 8% of patients undergoing this procedure

C – **T** although single vessel disease was the first indication for angioplasty, it can now be attempted for multi-vessel disease and also for more than one occlusion in the same vessel

D – **T** angioplasty is effective in these circumstances and is the method of choice in such patients

E – **T** this procedure should not be attempted without full cardiac surgical facilities readily available in case of dissection of the coronary artery or acute rupture (<5%): although some hospitals in London do perform PTCA without on-site cardiac surgeons, these facilities are close by in other hospitals

POST-MYOCARDIAL INFARCTION

81. A – **F** Dressler syndrome consists primarily of painful pericarditis usually 2 to 12 weeks after infarction while the shoulder–hand syndrome is characterised by a painful swollen left hand up to 7 months after infarction

B – **F** although the shoulder–hand syndrome is much more frequent in the left hand, it can sometimes involve the right arm also

C – **T** this may be associated with atrophy of the muscles of the left upper limb and flexion contractures of muscles also

D – **T** Dressler syndrome is thought to be due to an auto-immune antibody response to pericardial and myocardial antigens exposed to the immune system when infarction occurs

E – **F** Dressler beats are fusion beats occurring in ventricular tachycardia

82. A – **F** initially this was thought to be so, but their anti-arrhythmic properties are minimal and other mechanisms are thought to be responsible

B – **F** the Norwegian study was of timolol versus placebo [1] and showed a 16.8% v 10.4% reduction in mortality at a mean time of 17 months post infarction. This was the first convincing and adequately controlled trial of β-blockers in myocardial infarction

C – **T** the BHAT study [2], compared propranolol to placebo after acute infarction and showed a reduction in mortality from 9.5% to 7% at a mean of 24 months

D – **F** atenolol appears to prevent early death by reducing incidence of ventricular rupture, rather than preventing later death, as shown in the ISIS 1 trial [3]

E – **F** treatment should probably be continued indefinitely

[1] The Norwegian Multicentre Study Group. N Engl J Med. 1981;304:801–7.

[2] Beta Blocker Heart Attack Research Study Group. JAMA. 1982; 247:1707–14.

[3] ISIS 1 Research Group. Lancet. 1986;ii:57–65.

POST-MYOCARDIAL INFARCTION PROPHYLAXIS

83. A – **F** no adequate trials have been performed of anti-coagulation after myocardial infarction, although the Dutch '60-plus' study [1] showed that the stopping of warfarin, previously given for acute myocardial infarction, resulted in a higher fatality rate than if warfarin was continued

B – **T** ISIS 2 [2] amongst other studies has shown that 160 mg aspirin daily used alone or in conjunction with streptokinase reduced mortality after myocardial infarction

C – **T** the benefit of dipyridamole was no greater than that of aspirin, even when used in combination with aspirin [3]

D – **F** trials of numerous drugs (e.g. mexilitene, disopyramide) have all failed to show a reduction in mortality, even though they do suppress arrhythmias. It may be their pro-arrhythmic and negatively inotropic properties that have adverse effects on mortality

E – **F** the Anturane reinfarction study [4] initially suggested some improvement but when analysed on an 'intention to treat' basis, there was no difference in survival between the groups

[1] Sixty Plus Reinfarction Group. Lancet. 1980;2:989–94.
[2] ISIS 2 Collaborative Group. Lancet. 1988;2:349–60.
[3] Persantin–Aspirin Reinfarction Study Group. Circulation. 1980;62:449–61.
[4] Anturane Reinfarction Trial Research Group. N Engl J Med. 1980;302:250–6.

PRIMARY PULMONARY HYPERTENSION (PPH)

84. A – **F** PPH occurs predominantly in females (3/4 of cases)

B – **T** but only in African patients, and it is caused by schistosomiasis

C – **T** 10–30% of patients with PPH have Raynaud disease

D – **F** only 50% of patients with PPH diagnosed in life are found to have evidence of thrombo-embolic disease at autopsy

E – **F** the ventilation/perfusion scan is usually normal. Doing a scan in these patients may be dangerous because the large albumin aggregates used in the test may block off completely pulmonary arterioles already narrowed by the disease

QT SYNDROME

85. A – **T** the relationship with heart rate is similar to that in the normal ECG

B – **T** the shortening of the QT is probably the result of the increased sympathetic tone during exercise

C – **T** this occurs in the Jervell and Lange–Nielsen syndrome, the other features of which are syncope and a tendency to sudden death. It is a condition of childhood

D – **F** hypokalaemia prolongs the QT interval more and may facilitate the development of ventricular tachycardia

E – **T** a prolonged QT interval has been reported in intensive weight-reduction regimes involving liquid protein diets; it has also been recorded in patients with anorexia nervosa

RADIATION AND HEART DISEASE

86. A – **F** in the early days of radiotherapy, the heart was thought to be rarely involved, but this may have been due to inadequacy of proper reports. With recent advances in DXR techniques and concentration of radiation to the anterior mediastinum, e.g. for breast cancer, cardiac complications have been found to occur

B – **F** it is the pericardium which is most often affected resulting in effusion and tamponade in the short-term and constriction long-term

C – **F** radiation can damage the coronary arteries and result in infarction

D – **F** the incidence of coronary atherosclerosis as a complication is greater when irradiating the left breast

E – **F** there is a predilection for the left anterior descending artery and the proximal part of the right main coronary artery. This is probably due to the frequency of DXR treatment to the anterior mediastinum

RHEUMATIC FEVER

87. A – b incidence of carditis is 50%
B – a incidence of arthritis is 80%
C – c incidence of chorea is 10%
D – e incidence of permanent valve disease is 30%
E – d incidence of erythema marginatum is 5%

RHEUMATOID HEART DISEASE

88. A – **T** the usual manifestations of cardiac involvement are pericarditis and endocarditis
B – **F** pericarditis occurs in about 30% of patients with rheumatoid heart disease, and most of these have an effusion
C – **T** the mitral valve is the one most frequently affected in rheumatoid heart disease, with the aortic, tricuspid and pulmonary valves involved in that order
D – **F** the commonest ECG abnormality is first-degree block. LBBB may sometimes occur, as well as atrial fibrillation
E – **T** the incidence of significant coronary disease at autopsy in rheumatoid patients is 20%. The likely cause is arteritis

SARCOIDOSIS AND THE HEART

89. A – **F** the commonest cause of death from sarcoidosis in the UK is respiratory failure due to cor pulmonale as a result of pulmonary involvement. However, myocardial involvement is the main cause of death from sarcoidosis in Japan

B – T conduction disturbances are the commonest clinical presentation, and complete heart block is the most frequent manifestation, though bundle branch block is also common, RBBB more often than LBBB

C – F angina can occur in about 25% of patients with systemic sarcoidosis [1]. The precise cause is not known – it may be due to vasculitis, microvascular involvement or, very rarely, to direct involvement of the epicardial or intramyocardial coronary arteries by sarcoid

D – F a positive biopsy is obtained in only 50–60%, and then only if both left and right ventricles are extensively involved. Clinical suspicion should be roused in any patient with bilateral hilar adenopathy and clinical and/or ECG evidence of cardiac disease

E – T steroids are indicated in sarcoidosis with cardiac involvement and should always be tried. However, there is evidence that they may facilitate the development of ventricular aneurysm and this should always be kept under observation in a patient so treated

[1] Wait JL, Movahed A. Anginal chest pain in sarcoidosis. Thorax. 1989;44:391.

SYMPATHOMIMETICS

90. **A – T** although dopamine must be given through a central vein because of its irritant effects on smaller veins, dobutamine may be given through a peripheral line

B – T because it has no such effect, it is less likely to cause tachycardia than dopamine

C – F the myocardial nerve terminals do not release noradrenaline in response to dobutamine, although dopamine does cause its release

D – F dobutamine is the only inotrope that does not cause a severe tachycardia in usual doses

E – F both dopamine and dobutamine cause peripheral vasodilatation which is a β_2-receptor-mediated effect

TAKAYASU'S ARTERITIS

91. A – **T** antibodies are found to aortic wall, and there is also a relationship with HLA types. Other factors which may be relevant in the aetiology include streptococcal infection, tuberculosis and collagen disease

B – **F** females:males = 8:1

C – **T** Takayasu's original case described in 1908 was diagnosed on the basis of an arterio–venous retinopathy. More recent series have found retinal involvement in no more than 25%

D – **F** pulmonary involvement occurs in about 45% of patients

E – **F** the two conditions are easily distinguished by clinical examination. Although both conditions are diagnosed by finding reduced pulses in the limbs, in coarctation of the aorta the reduced pulses are in the legs, in Takayasu's arteritis the poor pulses are in the arms

VENTRICULAR ANEURYSM

92. A – **F** apart from trauma, ventricular aneurysms may develop as a result of myocardial sarcoidosis, syphilis (gumma formation) or rheumatic necrosis

B – **F** over 80% are found anteriorly near the apex and only 5–10% are located posteriorly

C – **T** 75% of the patients with LV aneurysms have triple vessel disease

D – **T** true ventricular aneurysm rarely ruptures, probably because it takes at least 6 weeks after infarction for the aneurysm to develop, and by this time fibrosis is well established before they are diagnosed. It is the pseudo-aneurysms developing soon after infarction which are prone to rupture, and they should be considered for aneurysmectomy as soon as possible after diagnosis

E – **T** the three commonest cause of heart failure are extensive myocardial damage following infarction, left ventricular aneurysm and mitral regurgitation due to papillary muscle dysfunction

VENTRICULAR SEPTAL DEFECT

93. A – **F** these areas of the septum are involved in 60% of cases, associated with atheroma of the anterior descending artery and full thickness anterior myocardial infarction

B – **T** only 20% of VSDs are in the posterior part of the septum and thus involve the mitral valve by infarction and rupture of the papillary muscles

C – **F** 40% patients who survive the acute phase of septal rupture develop aneurysmal dilatation of the remainder of the infarcted septum and ventricle

D – **T** 66% occur within 3 days of infarction and the rest within 7 days of onset. 1–3% of myocardial infarctions are complicated by VSD and they account for 1–5% of deaths in the peri-infarct period

E – **T** 25% are fatal within 24 hours of rupture and 50% are dead within 1 week. Less than 30% survive 2 weeks and only 20% are alive at 30 days. Without surgery, long-term survival is rare and early surgery is indicated

VENTRICULAR TACHYCARDIA

94. A – **T** short salvos require no treatment unless causing haemodynamic embarrassment. VT should be treated if at a rate of 120/min for >30 sec or >160/min for 15 sec

B – **F** a thump on the chest may work. DC conversion is required if the arrhythmia is rapid (>130) and continuous rather than paroxysmal – and is not the result of digoxin toxicity

C – **F** hypokalaemia is associated with VT, particularly in patients on long-term diuretics, and also with hypomagnesaemia; magnesium sulphate may be included in the treatment regime (10 ml of 50% $MgSO_4$ in 100 ml 5% dextrose given over 60 min for every 20 mmol potassium infused)

D – **F** although this is an option usually reserved for desperate situations: the bretylium tosylate is given as 400 mg in 5% dextrose over 10 min – it may however take 20 min to be effective and may cause serious hypotension

E – **T** drug treatment should be avoided as torsades de pointes may be drug-induced. It is best treated by correcting the potassium level, and stopping any drug that may prolong the QT interval (e.g. amiodarone); also by giving magnesium and sometimes by atrial pacing

95. A – **F** the insertion of a bipolar pacing wire in the high right atrium and the recording of the atrial ECG is of great use as the 1:1 relationship between P waves and the QRS complex confirms the supraventricular origin of the arrhythmia

B – **F** if the tachycardia complexes appear similar to the previous appearance of the bundle branch complexes, then supraventricular origin of the arrhythmia is established

C – **F** Rsr in V1 is characteristic of ventricular tachycardia, but rSR in V1 is a feature of supraventricular arrhythmias

D – **F** the deepest QS is in V4–5 in ventricular tachycardia. It is in left bundle branch block that the QS is deepest in the septal leads

E – **T** changing wave fronts (torsades de pointes) are a characteristic feature of ventricular tachycardia, usually associated with prolonged Q–T interval on the ECG